Breast Cancer:

NO ONE CHOSE
THIS JOURNEY

A Tribute

Breast Cancer:

NO ONE CHOSE
THIS JOURNEY

A Tribute

Fran Padgett

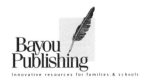

Bayou Publishing
Innovative resources for families & schools

Library of Congress Control Number:
ISBN-13: 978-1-886298-33-0

Printed in United States of America.

Artist notes regarding the series included in this book:

Other Side of the Mountain, created as a sequel to Moving On (published in *No One Wrote A Manual*), the images represent a traveler's encounters while traversing the Universe: the heavens, the earth, the weather.

Gift of Time, created in response to a research physician's successful treatment of a breast cancer patient who came to him with an expectation of 24 hours to live, and is still alive after 24 months. A gift of time. The series then expanded to recognize the spirit of more breast cancer patients traveling in search of their gift of time through medical treatment.

Weathervane is a trademark of Sunrise to Sunrise, Inc.

Bayou Publishing, 2524 Nottingham, Houston, TX 7005-1412.
www.bayoupublishing.com
(713) 526-4558

This book is dedicated to Esther Valdez, R.N., MammaCare Specialist.

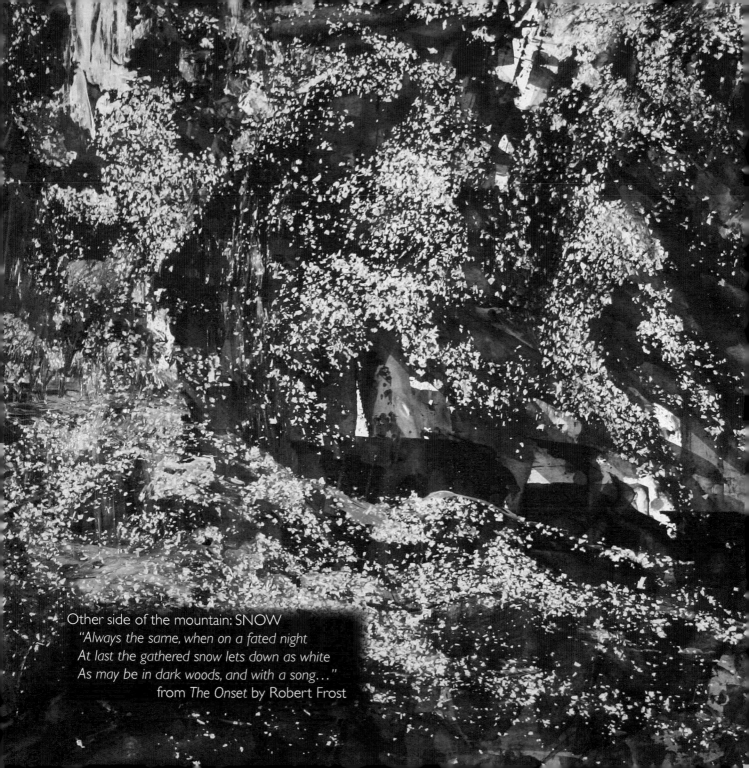

Other side of the mountain: SNOW
"Always the same, when on a fated night
At last the gathered snow lets down as white
As may be in dark woods, and with a song…"
from *The Onset* by Robert Frost

CONTENTS

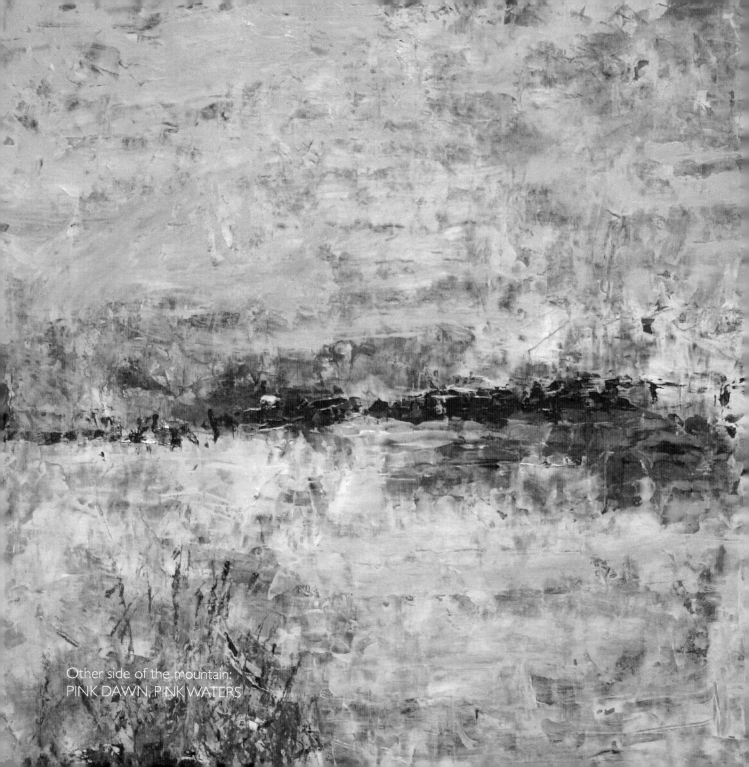

Other side of the mountain:
PINK DAWN, PINK WATERS

INTRODUCTION

No One Chose This Journey: The Gift Exchange

In your hands you hold a book capturing words and images of a most special gift exchange. It all began somewhat unintentionally at a professional convention in Galveston. I was sitting at the publisher's table signing copies of my previous work *Breast Cancer Recovery: No One Wrote a Manual,* when my agent introduced me to women who wanted to share with me their own stories. There was Amy, who was anxious to share the story of her mother-in-law Mozelle, a really tough lady from Timpson, Texas. After Amy came Deborah, her bravado not covering her fear. She was told by doctors only a week prior that she had an invasive ductal carcinoma.

With each passing week, as I attended gallery exhibits, civic luncheons, conventions across America, more and more "Amy's," and "Deborah's", fathers, husbands and sons, came up to talk to me. I've found it has become a most gratifying part of my unchosen journey to hear these breast cancer experiences, to be given favorite colors and snippets of life, sparking the creation of a painting I could dedicate to each one. Soon we saw the growing nucleus of a new project.

With these narratives, these vignettes, come glimpses of rare human strength, showing courageous decisions, and the spiritual beauty of these women. You may find yourself reading through tears, maybe your jaw clenched in frustration, or with a smile as you relate to a "really tough lady."

This is my tribute, my gift, to these brave ladies.

SPECIAL THANKS

Cindy Guire, Ecoversity, gifted artist with an exceptional graphic "eye"

Joanne Kirk, most trusted friend, confidante, person of outstanding varied skills and willingness to be frank and open

J. Julian Hewitt, art lover and art agent extraordinaire

Jennifer Shaeffer, intern, University of Houston, granddaughter of breast cancer survivor

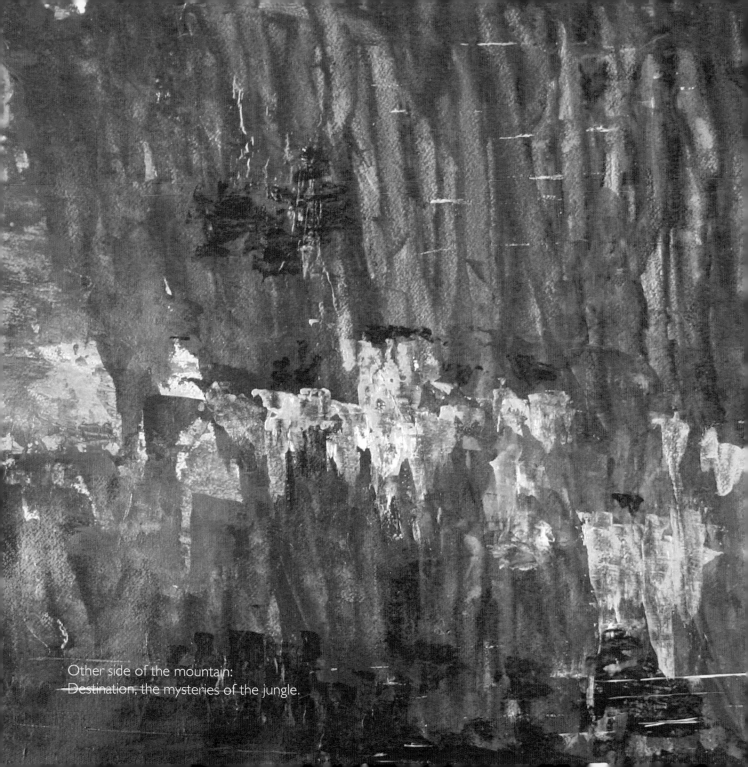

Other side of the mountain:
Destination, the mysteries of the jungle.

ACKNOWLEDGEMENTS

"*…I need a lending ear,*" began the letter from a lady who was caring for her beloved mother dying of breast cancer.

Dr. Sutton, are you psychic? Did you know when you asked if sometimes one of your new breast cancer patients could call me, that it could be the beginning of this book about those who are on the journey of breast cancer?

The sojourners I write about here are not your patients. Some may have gone years ago. Some are from Viet Nam, from Pennsylvania, from Arkansas, Mississippi, Michigan, Minnesota, Louisiana, or Texas – Amarillo to Timpson to Galveston. But in all of them you will recognize inspiring, incredible resilience, beauty and toughness.

An acknowledgement at the beginning of a book is where the author can say "thank you" to those who have been instrumental in making it possible. "Thank you" seems so inadequate Dr. Sutton, but those are the only words I know. I hope you like my new book.

— Fran Padgett

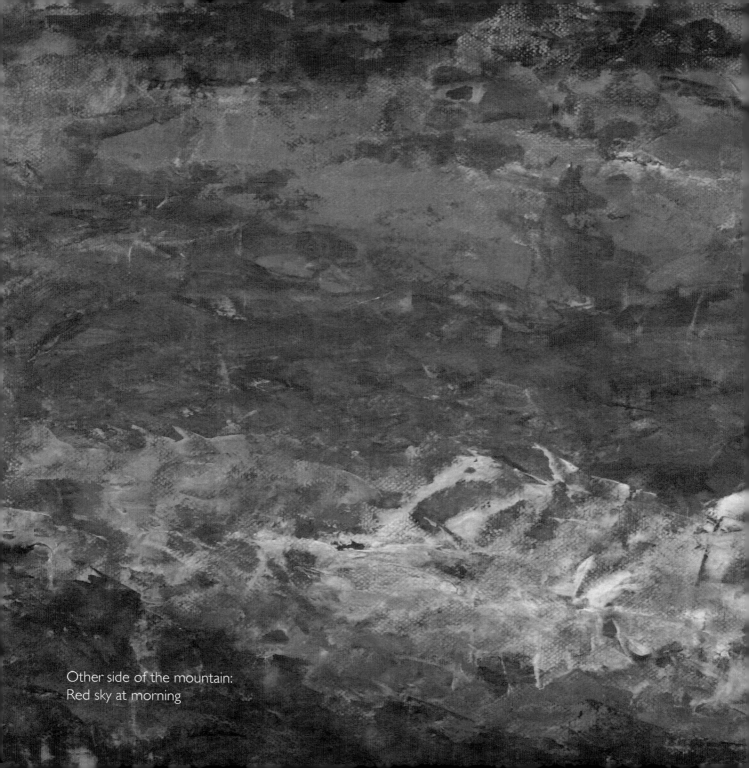

Other side of the mountain:
Red sky at morning

PROLOGUE:

ENTER ESTHER

The Breast Center at Houston Northwest Medical Center:

Esther quickly enters the conference room that has been decorated with flowers and pink ribbons. She has hurriedly changed out of her nurses' scrubs and now stands facing a semicircle of seated women who have been waiting for her arrival. The faces of these women reflect the spirit and strength exclusive to those who have heard the words 'breast cancer.' One has a newly installed chemo port on her chest wall, one has her arm connected to bags on mobile IV holders and has come down from the surgery floor of this breast center just to attend this gathering, three have pink caps to cover new baldness, most are barely concealing emotion.

Esther says, "Welcome," and once again begins the support group meeting with "no one chose this journey! We are here to help you … we will walk this walk with you."

Starting with the woman on her right, Esther asks each woman to tell us her name, when she was diagnosed, and to share any other information they would like. The first woman is very hesitant, softly saying only her name and that she was diagnosed a month ago. "Welcome," Esther tells her.

The next woman adds that she is a third grade teacher but is not able to work right now. "Welcome," Esther tells her, "we are glad you are here tonight."

One woman says, "And this is my granddaughter. She comes to support me because I'm alone now since my son is in the Marines in Iraq." "God bless you," Esther tells her, and everyone applauds.

The next woman is tearful. Her voice quivers, "I start my chemo tomorrow. I'm really scared." And Esther says, once again, "Welcome. No one chose this journey. We are here to help you – you can call us any time. We will walk this walk with you."

Esther had been an ICU and emergency room nurse for seventeen years. For seven months she and her sister kept a constant vigil at the bedside of their mother as she succumbed to cancer. She then answered an inner calling to "do something for women," and became a MammaCare Specialist.

Breast cancer has not chosen Esther. She travels this journey with her breast cancer patients because she chooses. And I, as one who was "chosen by breast cancer" am in awe of someone like Esther who tells us, "no one chose this journey; we are here to help you as you travel this road."

If we are lucky, we may all know a nurse like Esther.

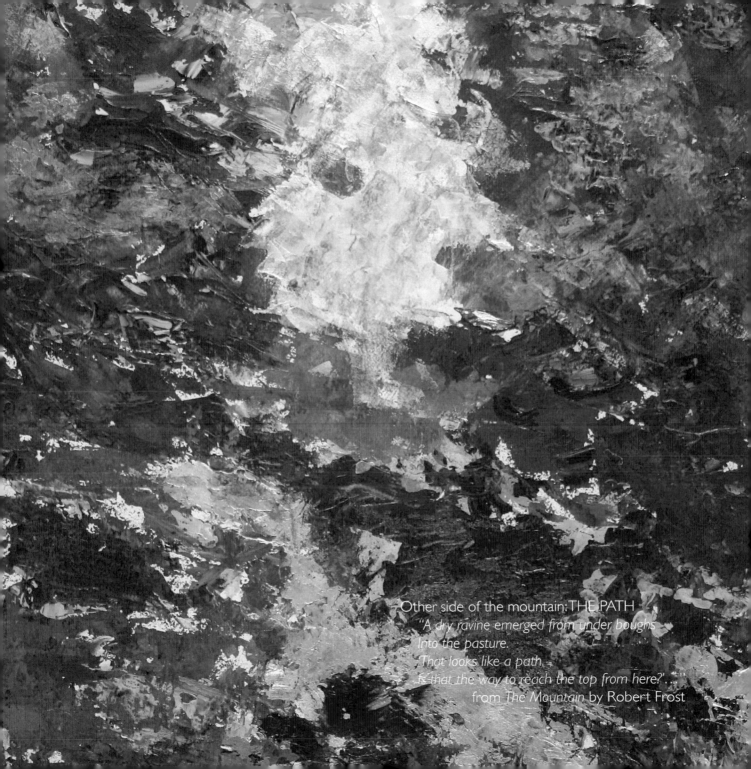

Other side of the mountain: THE PATH
*"A dry ravine emerged from under boughs
Into the pasture.
That looks like a path.
Is that the way to reach the top from here?"...*
from *The Mountain* by Robert Frost

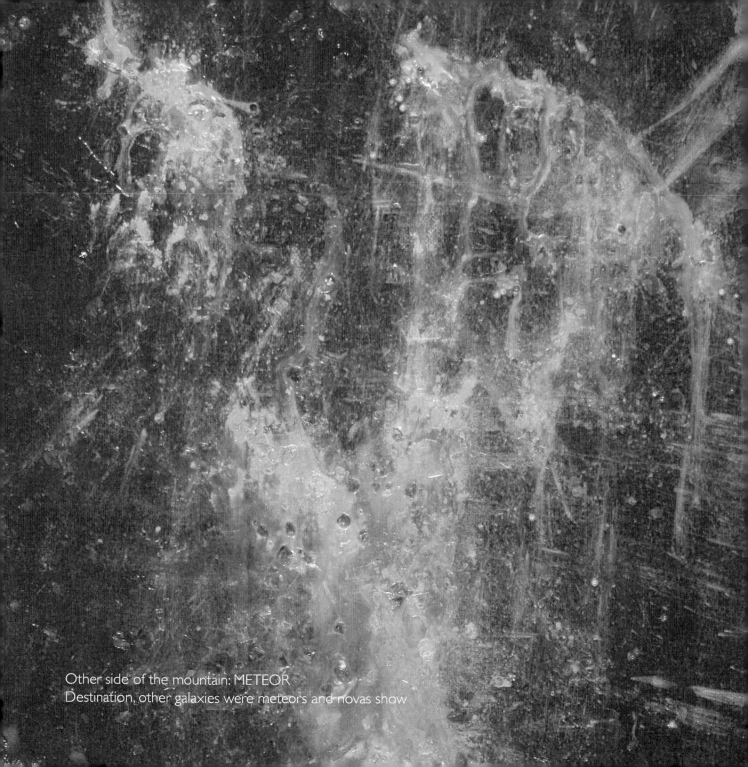

Other side of the mountain: METEOR
Destination, other galaxies were meteors and novas show

CHAPTER ONE

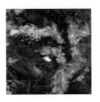

GALVESTON

Galveston, oh Galveston,
I still hear your sea winds blowing...I still hear your sea waves crashing
From Galveston Oh Galveston, *by Jimmy Webb*

Sunrise to Sunrise: Searching for Solitude

My journey begins. January 2nd.

The sun shines bright overhead as I drive the old highway to Galveston. Coming to the coastal plain, open and rugged in its way, is soothing. There is almost no traffic. Check in time at the resort is mid afternoon and I should arrive about that time. My mind's clock has stopped for a while so I don't think about what awaits in five more days...the surgeon's scalpels, the bright lights overhead in the operating room.

Because I have chosen to go where I can be alone for a few days, my family fears I have departed to end my life. They don't understand I am searching my soul for my strength to start a different life. I had previously dedicated my life to caring solely for my family. Now at this new destination, I must care for myself. I detest the thought that they might need to care for me.

The streets of Galveston are vaguely familiar; it was easy to find Seawall Boulevard where the San Luis Resort rises 16 stories above the boulevard, built on a manmade headland as hopeful protection from hurricane wind and tidal surges. The Gulf of Mexico lacks the Hollywood beauty of the Atlantic. The San Luis Resort is modest compared to those along the beaches of Miami, but every room faces east to see the sun rise over the sandy water.

A parking valet meets me and opens the car door. He smiles.

A bellhop takes my bags and escorts me to the registration desk. He smiles.

The young desk clerk finds my reservation in her computer and hands over the room key. She smiles.

Three people so far who do not know—to them I am just a woman who has traveled alone to watch the surf and sketch each sunrise.

All my family, my friends, my colleagues, my acquaintances both far and near, they all know. Here I will have three days—three blessed days and nights—alone where no one knows I have breast cancer; no questions I need to answer, no questioning glances I have to avoid, only blessed solitude with surf and sunrises.

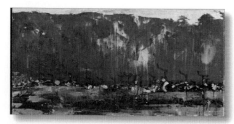 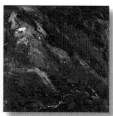 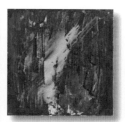 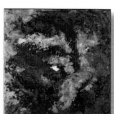

Other side of the mountain. Destination, Unknown waters

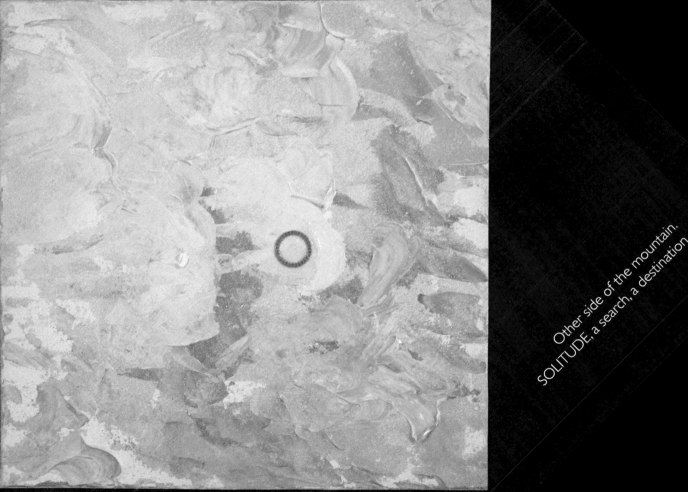

Other side of the mountain.
SOLITUDE, a search, a destination.

The Lady from Timpson, Texas
Galveston, oh Galveston, I am so afraid of dying…

The story of Mozelle who was born in Timpson, Texas, told by Amy, Galveston, Texas:

"We buried my mother in law 3 days ago. I want to tell you about her because she was uniquely special.

"She had breast cancer two times. But she died of other causes after she turned 92."

Amy continued to unfold the profile of a woman with spirit, beauty, elegance and toughness.

"She was diagnosed the first time in 1947. Her sister had succumbed to breast cancer a few years before. Mozelle's diagnosis struck fear into the heart of her family and her devoted husband.

"There was only one treatment for breast cancer in 1947: a radical mastectomy which stripped away not only breast tissue but the muscles from the chest wall, taking tissue and lymph nodes from the axilla; leaving pain and weakness across the chest and down the arm.

"When she was released from the hospital, Mozelle's husband took her to Galveston where she could regain strength along the beauty of the beach, listening to the waves, feeling the wind, watching the sun rise in glorious, soul-enriching colors.

"Returning home, Mozelle found an accordion and taught herself how to play the local music, strengthening her weakened arm muscle and toughening her chest wall now flat and scarred where once there was feminine softness. She would often refer to herself as 'O.S.S.' Initials that stood for 'one-sided sister.'

"A son was born, tenderly cuddled against O.S.S., the mother's bosom soft one side, flat hard surface the other. The infant took no notice, not knowing every other's mother's anatomy was different.

"As she grew older she stayed slender, she walked gracefully elegant, with her head high, her shoulders back. Her skin remained smooth, and like a porcelain doll, she looked lovely in pink.

"With caring spirit she volunteered at the hospital.

"Breast cancer was diagnosed again in 2002. This time the mastectomy was a 'modified radical,' leaving skin with tissue and one narrow scar. Fifty-five years have brought some advancements in breast cancer treatment. But still surgery. Still traumatic. Just less brutal than earlier in the 20th century. Her toughness was tested one more time.

"In 2003 Mozelle's secret dream to travel came true when her family presented a birthday gift of a 10 day cruise. She cried tears for happy. Well, not always so tough after all.

Image left and right:
Gift of time for Mozelle. Elegant. Tough.

"In 2005 Mozelle slipped away from this Earth and entered the peace of eternity, still beautiful, still elegant, still spirited. Still lovely in pink."

The town of Timpson, Texas lies between US 59 and an old railroad track. The rail line has been revitalized for freight to Mexico, but the town remains much as it must have looked a century ago – rural, agricultural – easy to envision Mozelle coming here to walk into stores and shops, to speak to friends and neighbors, to play the accordion at home for her family.

∽

Chemo Will Have To Wait

"…I am so afraid of dying…before I hear your sea winds blowin…
…before I ..hear your sea waves crashing…
…before I watch your seabirds flying in the sun…
…At Galveston, at Galveston."

Deborah approached my table where I was signing books at the convention center in Galveston. She seemed to hesitate. I asked her to please sit and visit with me for a few minutes. Her bravado not covering her fear, she opened the conversation with:

Image left and right: Gift of time for Deborah. Determined. Brave.

"My name is Deborah. I was born in Oklahoma but I was raised in Wisconsin. I like spring and summer best. I guess you could say I am a "warm weather person" especially now that I live in Amarillo.

"So far as I know there is no breast cancer in my family and I was astounded that an invasive carcinoma was found when I went for my routine mammogram last month.

"My doctor said the treatments will start with chemotherapy; I scheduled the first appointment to be when I get back to Amarillo.

"But I registered for this conference months ago because I have never been to Galveston and I wanted to see the Gulf of Mexico.

"I told the doctors that starting the chemo would just have to wait because I have this chance now to go to Galveston." Deborah paused, then continued, her voice very determined: "I told them 'I am going to Galveston and I AM going to see the Gulf of Mexico.'"

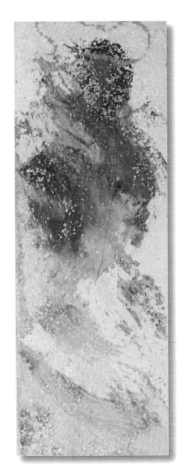

I told Deborah that I, too, had begun my breast cancer journey in Galveston. I hope, Deborah, that your journey will not be too difficult and that you return to Galveston sometimes, as I have, just to renew your love for this unique place along the Gulf of Mexico. And to celebrate your life.

Annie from Barbados
(What Price Vanity?)

Galveston, another time, another day:

Yesterday I stood at the shoe store sales counter. I was not in a hurry and watched while the only clerk, a woman whom I took to be about 60, finished ringing up my purchase. The only other customer, also a woman about 60, seemed not to be in a hurry as she waited to pay for practical oxford type shoes she had selected. .

We were three strangers, the only thing in common being the shoe store, and our age. The customer, I have named her Annie, made a comment directed mostly to the clerk, "Well, I am glad to be out of that doctor's office and that mammogram over.

The sales clerk made an acknowledging sound, like, "hmmmm." A few seconds went by before I said to Annie, "I'm glad to hear you took the time for a mammogram. I had cancer in both breasts at the same time. Mammograms are important." I rarely volunteer that information to strangers, but something about Annie made it seem I should.

Annie told us that her "Mummy" had ignored a breast lump for six years because, Annie said, "Mummy was very vain about her looks. When she finally did go to the doctor, the cancer was "all over her body." Annie motioned to her head and down her torso. It was too late. The Barbados doctor, where Mummy lived, performed first one mastectomy, then later a second mastectomy. But when Mummy finally came to New York for treatment, the physician who saw her told Annie that Mummy was already "a dead person walking around."

Annie closed her eyes, took a deep breath and said, "I have this large lump." With her right hand she indicated the side of her left breast. "I will have the doctor's report tomorrow."

Her fears were now revealed: Her own lump; her own mother's experience. "Mummy died in 1994. She suffered horribly."

To myself, I said, "Annie, I have heard those exact words before."

Annie looked at my card. "If the doctor's report is not good news, I will be calling you."

"I will be glad to talk to you," I assured her as I left the shoe store. Maybe I will hear from Annie. If I don't, I will hope it is because she has good news right now before Christmas, and she only remembers me as she checks her breasts.

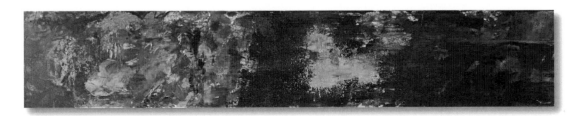

Image above and left: Gift of time in blue for "Annie" Island of fear.

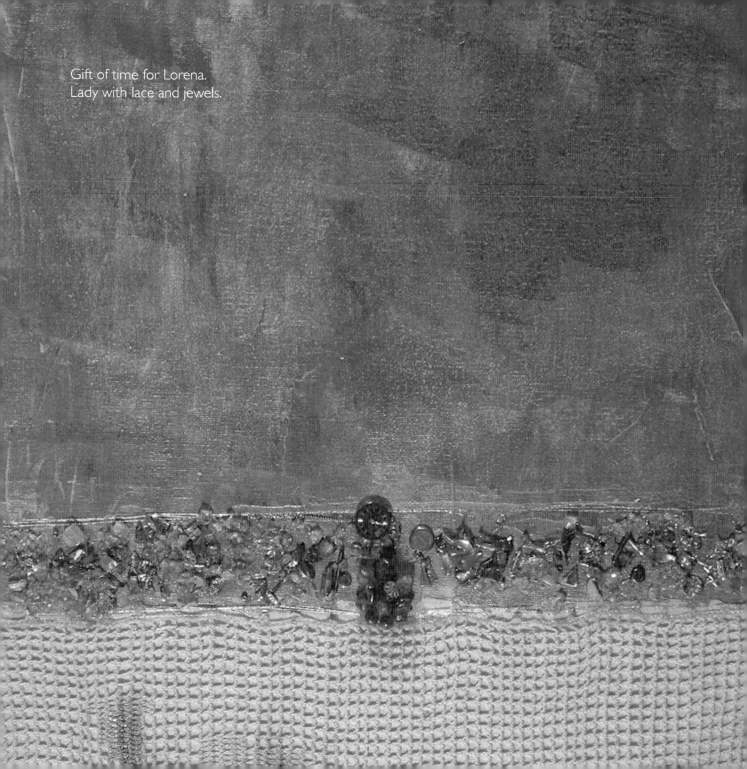

Gift of time for Lorena.
Lady with lace and jewels.

CHAPTER TWO

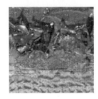

BEAUTIFUL SPIRIT

The best and most beautiful things in the world cannot be seen, nor touched....but are felt in the heart." —Helen Keller

Sometimes There Are Miracles

Eveline's exquisite beauty is like that of angel paintings Her story is below.

"Slowly I opened my eyes, still half asleep. It was Thanksgiving morning and my first waking thought was, I am alive, I am alive. Tears streamed."

Breast cancer came at 38. A gloomy prognosis. Immediate and aggressive chemotherapy started. The newest, latest and hopefully the most effective, from A to Z. And devout prayers from friends and family.

"I went to see the oncologist yesterday. She said, 'Eveline, I honestly did not expect that I would see you today.'"

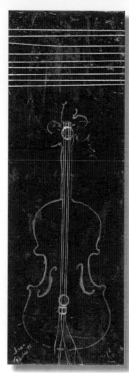

Sometimes there are miracles.

A lapse of a few months, then the testing once again. There is still cancer showing. Once again, a few more months of chemotherapy. Same drugs; different drugs. And the devout and fervent prayers of family and friends.

More than a year of chemotherapy. Eveline's beautiful skull left uncovered to skip the discomfort and inconvenience of caps or wigs. Her face pale and fragile belying inner strength—inner strength to endure the treatments and face the fear.

More tests. Mastectomy is now in order. Plus the benevolent grace of the Divine Providence.

Thanksgiving time again. Eveline writes:

"Dear all, Just returned from the doctor's office where I heard the most beautiful words. I am in complete remission. I am overjoyed and celebrating. Thank you for all your love and prayers. God has answered in a mighty way!"

Sometimes there are miracles!

But sometimes miracles don't give us a lot of time and must be measured in small gifts…like taking a long-awaited cruise.

Christmas time, same year. Eveline writes:

Dear all,

After my PET scan and other various tests, the results showed some cancer in my left side. The great news is it is nowhere else and I am so thankful for that. I just feel God's protection. The doctor will determine how to schedule chemo

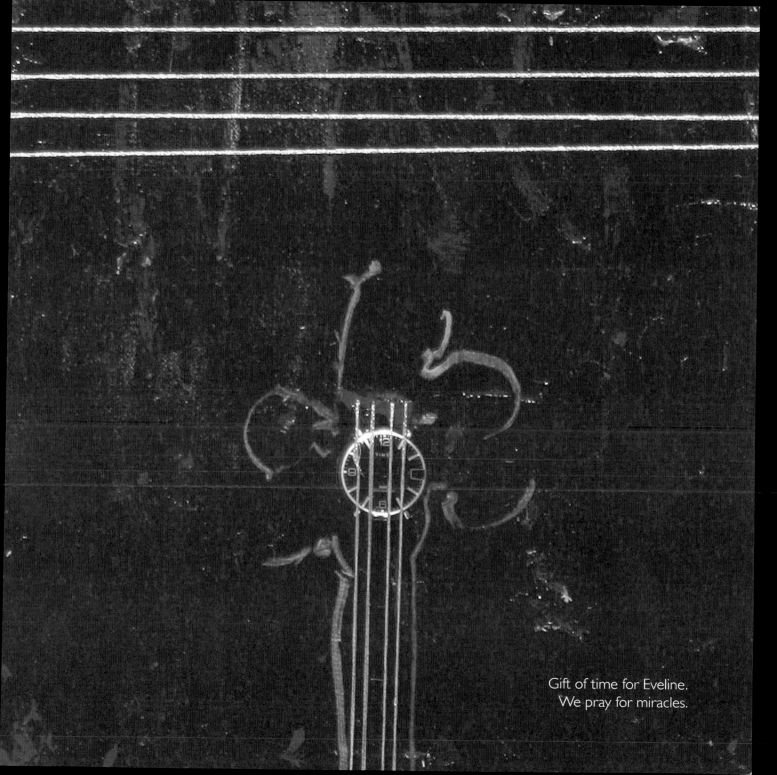

Gift of time for Eveline.
We pray for miracles.

so I'll see her again next week. The girls took it pretty hard (lots of tears) even with our reassurance. I get to keep working and Chris and I get to take our long awaited cruise at the beginning of February so I feel great. I get to enjoy life with my precious family. Thanks for your continual prayers. I am joyful in hope, patient in affliction and faithful in prayer: Romans 12:12. Thanks and love, Eveline.

Next letter (dated in June) Eveline writes:

Hi family and friends. My new tests were not exactly what I had hoped. No new growth but also no decrease so chemo continues. On the bright side, chemo now is a pill versus injection. One a week until after the beginning of July then another will be added. The wait is just to accommodate vacation plans. I will also get hair !!!!! Yeah, how exciting. I am optimistic and KNOW God has not completed the work He has begun in me yet. I'm patiently waiting! Thanks and love, Eveline.

Next letter (dated July), Eveline writes:

I had a check up on Friday. Two weeks of the new chemo done. The tumors are already smaller and the doctor is very pleased. God is blessing me again. The first week was a breeze, just a lot of pills to take. Week two was much tougher. I'm having trouble with my skin and lips cracking. Also a few other side effects. I have been resting a lot though and am relieved not to be going back to work. I'm not at all surprised now why the doctor said "no." As always, thanks for your prayers. Eveline

Next letter (August) Eveline writes:

Hi all. I just got home late today from a six-day stay at the hospital. I am so glad to be home!!!! I now think I have the most beautiful house in the world and am so thankful for the TLC I received at Chris' hospital [Eveline's husband Chris is a nursing supervisor at Houston Northwest Medical Center].

I won't do any chemo or meds until I see my doctor next Wednesday to help recover from the dehydration, etc. The doctor is testing for an enzyme some people have that responds negatively to one form of the chemo I take (xeloda). I am praying I don't have it so I can continue the Tykerb too because at this point the two drugs are approved together and Tykerb hasn't been tested with anything else. (I think all that is right, very confusing info…). I had a great reduction from the first round so just praying it was a tough first round and all that is over. So please continue your prayers for me and that I can continue this chemo. Thanks, Eveline.

Dear Eveline, I write:

From all your friends, we continue to pray for you and for miracles.

Champagne With Dee

Invitations were telephoned to a few close friends.

Champagne was delivered and chilled in silver buckets of ice.

Crystal glasses were set on silver trays, pink napkins tied with ribbon were stacked at the edge.

Lights were all dimmed except the one over the mirror.

The guest of honor sat calmly in the designated chair.

Her hostess turned down the music, poured the champagne, walked around to the guests who each took a glass and pink napkin.

"Let us have a toast." Champagne glasses tipped toward each other and touched edges with a musical ping.

"Here's to Dee."

"Cheers, Dee".

"Good luck."

The hostess stood behind Dee, raised her scissors and comb, and without flourish began removing Dee's short, wavy dark hair.

In minutes, Dee's bald head glowed from the light over the mirror.

Then the ladies raised their glasses, a final round of toasts to Dee.

"We love you, Dee."

Only a woman with such great inner strength would provide a celebration for her closest friends to be a part of the loss of her hair before her first chemotherapy. Making it easy for them to watch her become bald. What a friend!

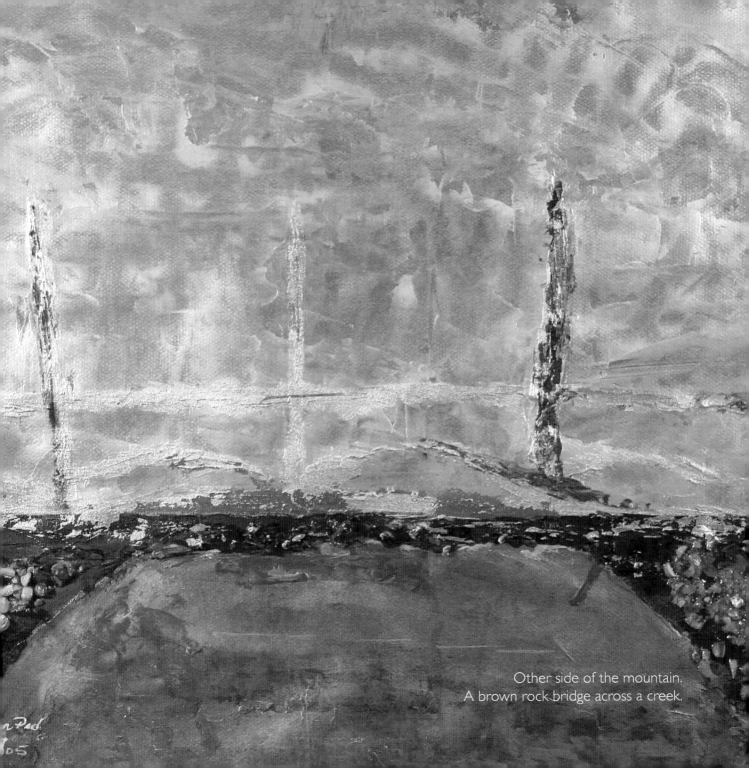

Other side of the mountain.
A brown rock bridge across a creek.

Judy, the painting Judy, the Family Caretaker

Christmas Eve I wrote,

Dear Diane,

When you first told me about your sister Judy's breast cancer, we spoke of a Gift of
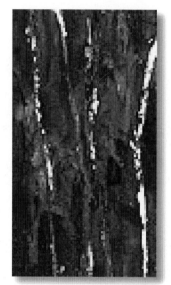
Time painting to be dedicated to her. As you talked, the colors which kept flashing in my mind were cream and ivory. When you called saying her favored colors were beige, tan and camel I wasn't surprised – cream and ivory, beige, tan and camel are all shades of same color family.

Then Diane, while I thought about how her painting would develop, intuition told me to use heads and stems of wheat as symbols of life's sustenance. To complete the composition, I would incorporate natural twine and blended fibers for texture.

A few days later when we met over lunch, you shared with me that Judy is a kind, and generous person – the one who is "always there" to take care of her family – making the wheat symbol just right. And, you told me, she is a skilled seamstress and upholsterer – making the selection of twine and fibers as reminiscent of her work.

This was a painting that just "came together easily." As you view and absorb the nuances of this composition I anticipate that you will see and feel more and more of the sister you love.

— My best and warmest regards.

Judy, her Story

Christmas Eve three years later came this letter from Diane:

Dear Fran,

It has been three years since Judy was diagnosed with breast cancer and I think of her everyday. Her life has seen a lot of changes I want to share with you.

Judy and I are the closest in age of all our family of nine; three were older and four were younger. We grew up in the country near Embarrass, Wisconsin, along the Embarrass River. Our house did not have running water and it was the daily morning chore for me and Judy to bring in the water from the well and the fuel oil for the cook stove and heater before we went to school. Probably this sounds like a life of hardship, but we didn't think so. I remember our childhood as lots of good times. In the winter we could go out sledding and skating when the river was frozen. In the summer we played kids' yard games like tag and "red rover." Especially I remember swimming in the Embarrass River because the water was clear all the way to the bottom and in most places not very deep, except for under the bridge.

After we were grown came the greater hardships for Judy. She was the one of us who cared for our older sisters and often their

Image left and right: Gift of time for Judy. Generous. Ever kind.

19

children when they developed different cancers. Our brother, the only boy in our family, committed suicide. It was inexplicable to all of us and it was mostly left to Judy to console our parents. Then Judy's younger daughter developed bone cancer and died when she was only 23, leaving two small children. Again, a life's circumstance where Judy was the one to whom the rest of her family looked for their comfort and strength.

Judy's work at the furniture upholstery company took a lot of physical strength but she was proud of her skill and worked there 35 years, even through the breast cancer treatments along with two other women working there who also had been diagnosed with breast cancer.

The day Judy went with her husband to the doctor's office to be told that her routine mammogram revealed breast cancer was the same day her husband's father died. Once again Judy faced what sometimes seems like more than her fair share of life's hardships.

But across these past three years since breast cancer, life has changed for Judy. Things are "easier." She said she has made it a priority to focus on the important. She and her husband have retired and they travel sometimes. The time she can spend with their five grandchildren is special and happy. She has come to visit me and I have traveled to Wisconsin to visit with her.

Even though it would seem that a diagnosis of breast cancer would be the ultimate hardship in a life filled with hardships, it has actually been the beginning of an easier phase in her life. And she is grateful.

Thank you for the painting, Fran, and thank you for caring. Hugs, Diane.

Corry's Mom: "Bye-Bye Cleavage"

River Oaks Bookstore, Houston

The bookstore manager was turning the key in the lock to close the store at the end of the day when he saw Corry hurriedly approaching. He stopped locking and held the door open for her. She walked quickly to my table. She was pretty, and petite, her smile open and friendly. I guessed before she told me that she was a school teacher. I had not packed away my book signing materials and was happy to meet with a woman who was the last on this afternoon to request a book.

She sat across from me and said, "Would you write your message to my Mom? Her name is Pat. She is going to have a mastectomy day after tomorrow. She lives in Minneapolis and I can't be there with her. She is having the mastectomy because last week she had a lumpectomy. The lumpectomy surgery did not result in 'clear margins.' It was disappointing news but she is strong."

"I have three younger sisters, Annie, Julie and Hallie. They live close to Mom and they will be at the hospital with her. I talked to them yesterday. They told me that they will stand around her bed before she goes to the operating room to give her hugs and kisses."

Corry smiled and her eyes sparkled. "Then they said they are going to sing "Bye-Bye Cleavage" to the tune of "Bye- Bye Blackbird."

Smiles and gentle humor, as only daughters can share.

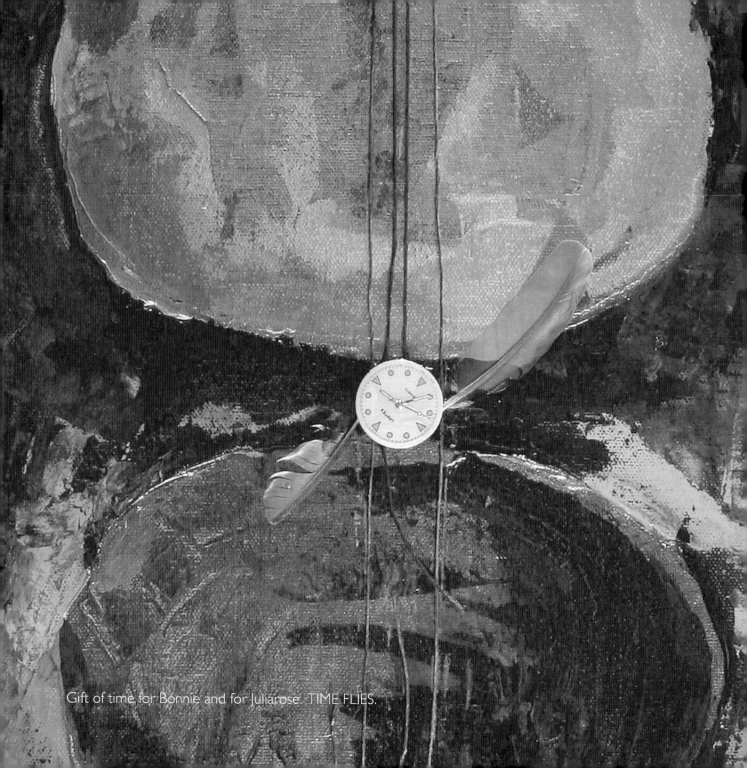

Gift of time for Bonnie and for Juliarose. TIME FLIES.

CHAPTER THREE

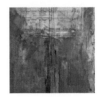

AWESOME STRENGTH

"Women are strong, even when they think they have no strength left."
—Author Unknown

Brave. Courageous. Proud.

From the newspaper eulogy for Virginia written by her friend George Hazard: "Bravery we define as advancing toward a monster unafraid. Courage we define as advancing toward a monster despite being afraid." I further define Virginia, a woman of awesome strength:

She picked the day she would die.

She loved dancing and riding, living and laughing.

She loved camellias and studied them.

She loved talking to people, her voice a husky Southern accent.

She loved politics and working on the City Council.

She loved her grandkids, making life and learning fun for them.

She loved her husband and nursed him through his final illness.

She said no to breast cancer treatments the second time it came.

She was brave, she was courageous, she was proud.

The Challenge Bike Ride of Bonnie J.

Tour de France:

Beginning point and finish line	Eiffel Tower, Paris, France
2,178 miles	21 days
Record time	86 hours 17 minutes 28 seconds by Lance Armstrong

Race Across America

Beginning point	Oceanside, California
Finish line	Atlantic City New Jersey
3,000 miles	14 days

First Texas team won in the team division 2005

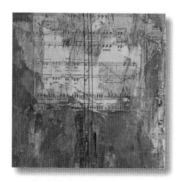
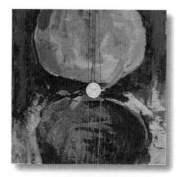
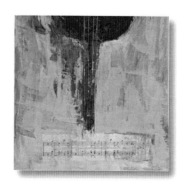

Bonnie's Challenge Bike Ride

Beginning point:	Bonnie's home in a north Houston subdivision
Finish line:	The Breast Center
14 miles	Time not clocked
Date:	March 23, 2006

"I thought I might have to stop to rest two or three times, but I didn't. I rode the 14 miles without stopping. The wind was blowing across my face. I think it was the wind created by my whizzing along at the edge of the curb. Friends offered to drive me. They didn't understand that this ride was my challenge to myself.

"Someone said a challenge bike race is one with no winners. But I won. I rode these 14 miles to my sixth and last chemotherapy treatment. I won."

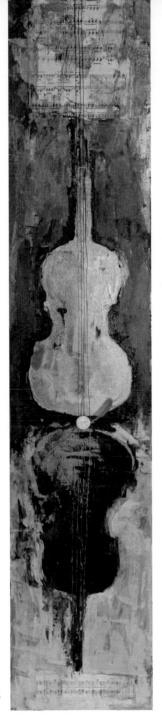

Image left and right: Gift of time for Bonnie and for Juliarose. TIME FLIES

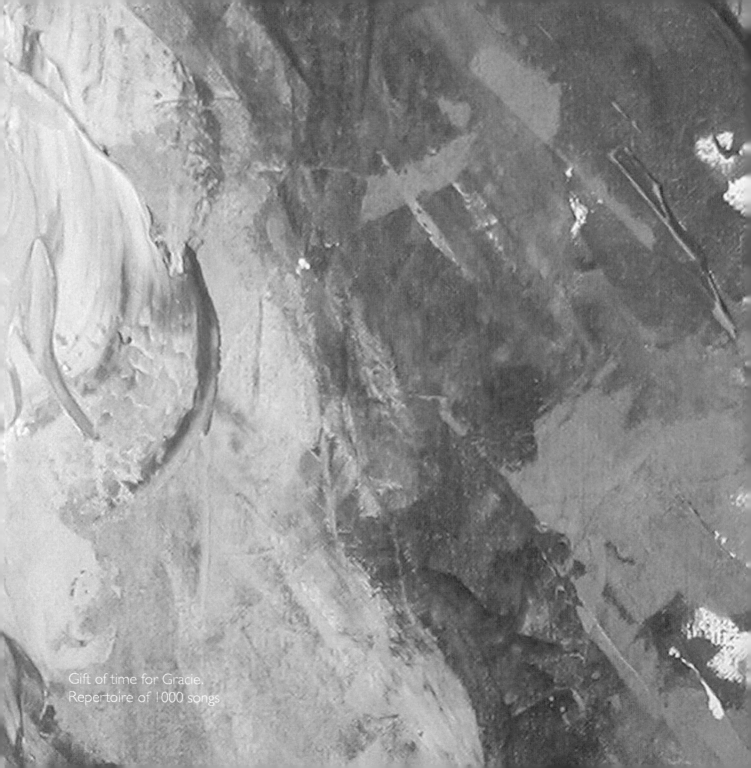

Gift of time for Gracie.
Repertoire of 1000 songs

CHAPTER FOUR

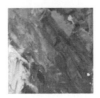

OVER AND OVER.
AND OVER AGAIN.

Breast cancer isn't always just one time…you are treated…then you are well and you go on with your life. Breast cancer sometimes recurs – sometimes after 27 years, like Gracie. Sometimes 3 times, like Jimmie Sue.

You never really forget this. It lurks in the back of your mind even though you stay busy and act like breast cancer is a thing in your past that you will never have to face…

AGAIN

Grace Anne: The Voice of an Angel; The Face of a Star

Memorial City Mall, Houston:

I watched Gracie as she sat on a tall stool in front of the stage. The television camera crew circled about her with lights, and the morning program host holding a microphone listened on his headset for his cue from the downtown studio signaling that they were ready to start the first segment of our live broadcast for a "Gift of Time" breast cancer fundraising event.

She seemed totally at ease like the accomplished, beautiful singer and actress she is. Totally at ease even though she would soon appear on the live morning television program with her head chemo-bald for the camera. A hairstylist waited to cover her evenly shaped skull with a blonde wig for the television audience. The crew and the host were all obviously admiring her beauty and confidence to be on a live television program with a chemo-bald head. While she waited to be the star of the morning show, she softly sang from her lifetime repertoire of a thousand or more songs.

New Orleans, early in the 1940's:

Grace Anne's life began with a prayer. Sarah Josephine traveled from Waco, Texas, to New Orleans where she prayed at the Shrine of St. Anne. She desperately yearned for children and grieved that all her babies did not make it to full term birth. She promised St. Anne that if she could be blessed with a child, the baby would be named for her.

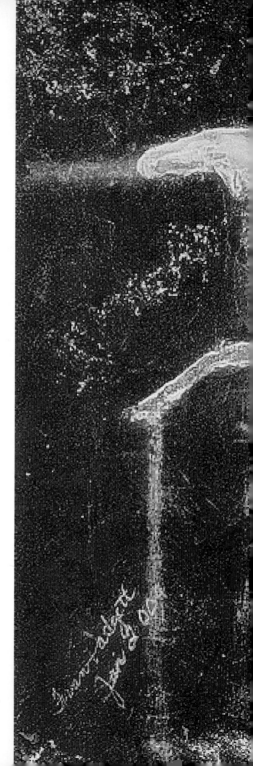

Other side of the mountain. Over the Milky Way. Destination, the stars.

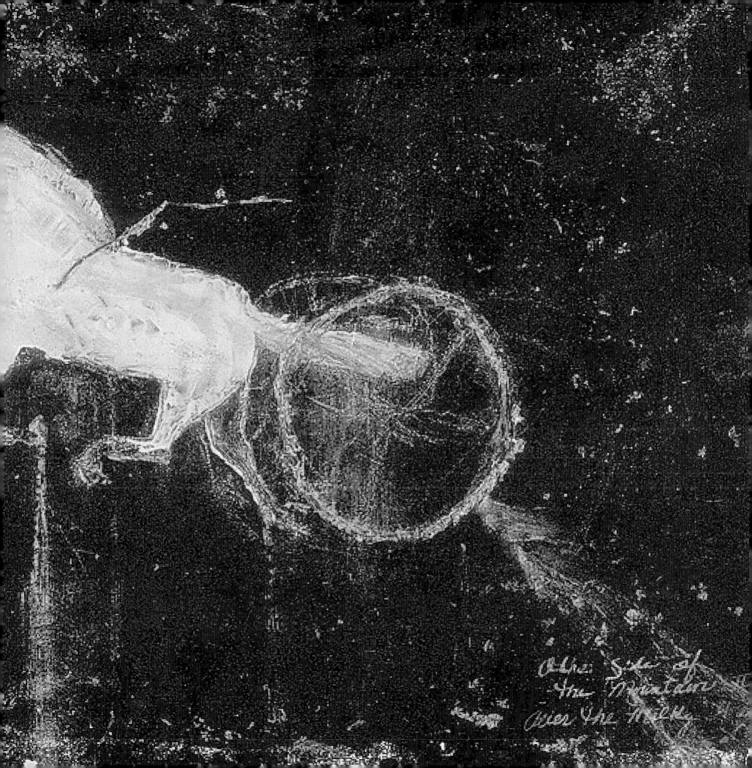

Other side of
the Mirror
over the Milky

Sarah Josephine returned to Waco where her prayer was answered when an exquisite infant was born. Keeping the promise, the baby was named Grace Anne. Grace means Anne – Anne means Grace.

St. Anne blessed her namesake with curly hair, angelic face and natural musical talent.

"Starting when I was 3 years old, I stayed at my parents restaurant while they worked, and I sat on the diner bar and sang for the customers. When I was five, my parents took me to Los Angeles because they believed I was 'the next Shirley Temple.'"

St. Anne gave Gracie a protective shield for surviving catastrophes.

"I have spent my life 'dodging bullets.' When I was seven I barely survived an acute hemorrhage after a routine tonsillectomy. When I was ten, the city of Waco was struck by a devastating tornado that destroyed most of the downtown, including my parents' restaurant. Another weather 'bullet' was Hurricane Allison coming to Houston. Another health 'bullet' was a staph infection that developed as a result of heart surgery.

"And of course, now I have had two 'episodes' of breast cancer. The first was when I was 33. I had noticed the lump the first time when I was 24. I went to a doctor who said, with no mammogram, no biopsy, 'oh, it is nothing, don't worry about it.' Of course it was hard for me to not worry and over the next several years I would go to doctors to have it checked. When I was in Europe I had a mammogram in Germany. A doctor in Amsterdam said, 'it is nothing to worry about.' Mammogram again in Zurich. Again I was told: 'nothing to worry about. I guess you could say I had 'cancer-phobia' – almost a hypochondriac – it is too hard to not worry about a breast lump that is obvious and growing. It was seven years from the first time the lump was showing to the first diagnosis.

"The second diagnosis was after 27 years of remission. Both times the surgery was a lumpectomy. The first time was followed by radiation which affected my heart. The second time there was divided opinion about undergoing chemo but I decided to start chemo."

St. Anne also blessed Gracie with intelligence, stamina, and talent for a variety careers.

"Of course there were acting and modeling classes. I was always in front of an audience. I went to New York City when I was nineteen, and I worked five part-time singing jobs while trying out

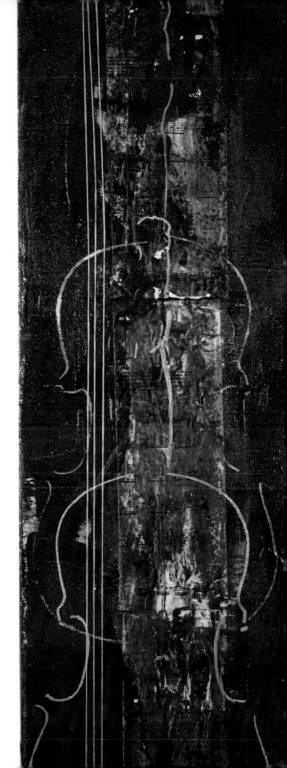

for play parts for the Broadway stage. At every audition I was told I really had talent and if the role hadn't already been filled I would have been 'perfect' for it. After four years I returned to Houston and became one of the first woman stock brokers in the city. I was good at it during the 'good times' but I would NEVER go back to it now. And now, I sing — my band and I now perform at gigs but only the ones we truly enjoy."

Houston Junior League, 2007, "Think Pink" a luncheon to raise funds for breast cancer endeavors:

Once again I watched Gracie perform. This time her head was no longer chemo bald. A short and shiny, wavy, blonde cap accented her perfect skull and movie star face. "Breast cancer gave me a sense of empowerment, like giving myself permission to do things like going blonde. And after the chemo bald, to leave my hair very short. So short I can cut it myself."

This performance was obviously a "gig" that Gracie truly enjoyed. With all her heart and soul and with only a pianist as accompaniment, she sang the story of her breast cancer journey. Opening with "On a Beautiful Day Like Today," then giving her audience smiles with personal revelations of bargaining with doctors; soon came chills with "I Will Survive," and tears, with her deep curtsy, a closing tribute of immense gratitude to her husband, Robert; and their daughter Sarah Jessica seated front row.

Lastly bows and kisses to her audience who were on their feet clapping for the inspiration and love from St. Anne through the voice of her namesake, Grace Anne.

Jimmie Sue (Times 3)

Jimmie Sue B., nee Malone, always dreamed to see Ireland, the land of her ancestors, her heritage.

The Irish have a beauty like no other in the world, beautiful faces, spiritual graces, lively, fun, tragic and strong, all at once. This island of fables and fairies holds a magnet to draw them to return, even if only once in life. And even if only after enduring breast cancer three times.

Jimmie's first realization of a lump in her left breast was on a fourth of July, she was in her twenties, married, the mother of a son and a daughter. What a scare! The treatment this time was a lumpectomy, followed by radiation, followed by chemotherapy.

Twenty years went by. Jimmie Sue was now the mother of one more son. Her daughter and both sons are now adults. A lump is discovered in her left breast once again. This time the treatment is a mastectomy followed by chemotherapy.

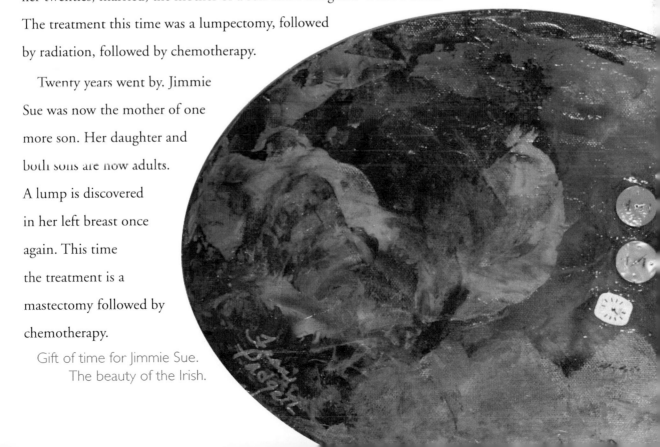

Gift of time for Jimmie Sue.
The beauty of the Irish.

Five more years go by. Now a lump in her right breast! This time the treatment is another mastectomy followed by chemotherapy. Jimmie Sue's family now includes grandsons and granddaughters who shared her dream to travel the bewitching island of Ireland.

One year ago, Jimmie Sue called me, excited, thrilled. "I have my Ireland tickets! My granddaughter Kathy is traveling with me. She is young and she can drive on the "wrong side of the road."

Jimmie Sue continued, "We will spend 3 full weeks. We will see the Malone family ancestral home. I will send you the pictures when I get back."

≈

Mothers and Daughters: What Are the Odds?

Within a year, a mother and two daughters have each been diagnosed with breast cancer. This story told by Anita, the third diagnosis.

"My sister, Pam, received the diagnosis on June 3rd in 2003. Isn't it amazing how we now just say "The Diagnosis" and we all know we refer to breast cancer.

"Our mother, Fern, was diagnosed in September 2003. That diagnosis was handed to us, her daughters, because she was already in advanced care for Alzheimer's. We did try to tell her but there was no understanding in her face

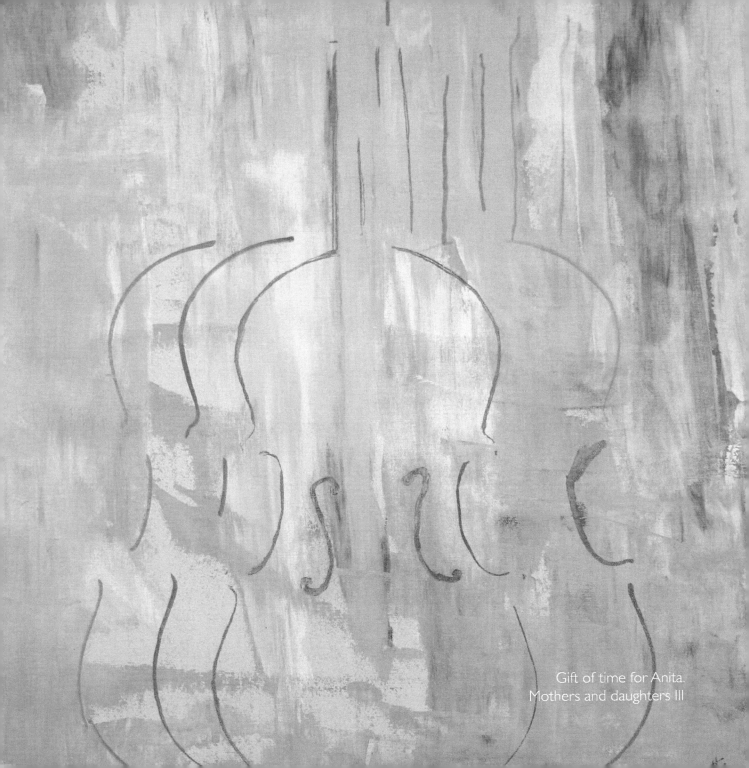

Gift of time for Anita.
Mothers and daughters III

or eyes. My sisters and I agreed that Mother's treatment should be limited to a mastectomy. She did not understand that either, why her chest was now lopsided.

"I received The Diagnosis on June 3rd, 2004; one year to the day after my sister Pam. But this time, The Diagnosis, for me was more than breast cancer because the tests revealed lymphoma. Treatments have been on-going and difficult. Now I am taking an anti-cancer drug. The side effects are very uncomfortable. I try to keep working and I come to the office at least 3 or 4 days a week even if I only stay for half the day.

"Of the three of us, I believe deep down in my heart, that it will be I who will die from the cancer. I don't know when, I don't think about it a lot and I don't fear it so much.

"One day my husband told our friends, 'We are going to our chemo appointment tomorrow.'

"Then he said to me, 'I hope you didn't mind my saying 'we.'

"I told him, ok, as long as you realize that this cancer is only about me. I am the one with lymphoma. I am the one with breast cancer."

"...Need A Lending Ear..."

...was the subject line from an email sent to me after Eryn read a Houston Chronicle article about me and my quest for breast cancer research. I have included her email here almost complete and verbatim...

"Hello Fran,

My name is Eryn. My mother's name is Shannon – she is currently going through her third mishap of breast cancer. Her first diagnosis was in 1991 and she elected to undergo a lumpectomy followed by radiation. She was in remission until 2004 when she found out she had to face her worst fear once more. She discovered the new lump by self-exam, that was again diagnosed cancer (lobular). At the time of diagnosis it was at stage 3 C, Hr Negative and it was in her lymph nodes. Treatment this time was a mastectomy followed by chemotherapy and radiation. Then she needed physical therapy for lymphedema in her left arm.

"During this past year pain developed in her tailbone and hips. Oncologists checked to see if the cancer had spread and 'lone and behold' [sic] the cancer had gone to her bones. She has just now started chemotherapy again and a bone strengthening medication. Since the cancer is Hr negative there are only some treatments she can be on, we've been told.

Gift of time for Shannon.

37

"I was wondering if in the research you are supporting if the few in my Mom's type of case could also one day find a cure. I feel so hopeless right now. I will nurse my Mom day and night and take care of her through her battle. I love her with all my heart and I thank God for her good days we may have."

After Eryn's mother passed away, Eryn shared with me that caring for her mother was a life changing experience and that she now wanted to become a nurse and an advocate for breast cancer research. I introduced her to Esther. Esther has now become Eryn's mentor while Eryn is enrolled in college to pursue a degree in nursing.

Eight Sisters and the Mysterious Double Line

Diane and I have been friends for ten years but lately we don't get to see each other as often as we wish. Sometimes we meet after work for a few sips of wine and conversation. Our first "let's catch-up" subject is always news of our families. Diane almost always would tell me about a sister's cancer diagnosis, or treatments or post-treatment condition, or of a sister's child or sadly, grandchild battling cancer and losing. She always referred to each of them as "my sister."

"Diane," I finally said one day, "tell me today about your sisters. How many are there, and which ones have the cancer or children or grandchildren with cancer?"

I started taking notes. From oldest to youngest I wrote:

Lyle ("Tootie")

Marion

Shirley

Judy

Diane

Sandra

Barbara

Sherry

From Lyle down thru Judy were the cancers; from Diane down thru Sherry no cancers, which prompted me to draw a double line between Diane and Judy. When Diane and I looked at my scribbled notes, we were struck by the mystery of it. Does it make Diane "next in line" to be diagnosed? Or does it foretell the good health fortune of the four youngest?

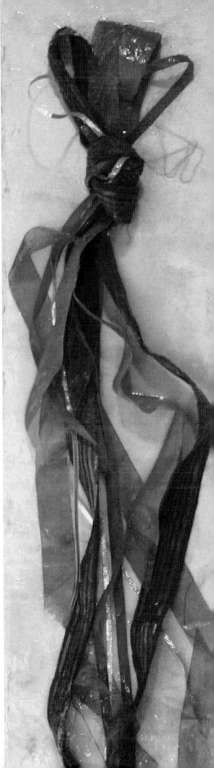

RIBBONS. Speak their language in code.

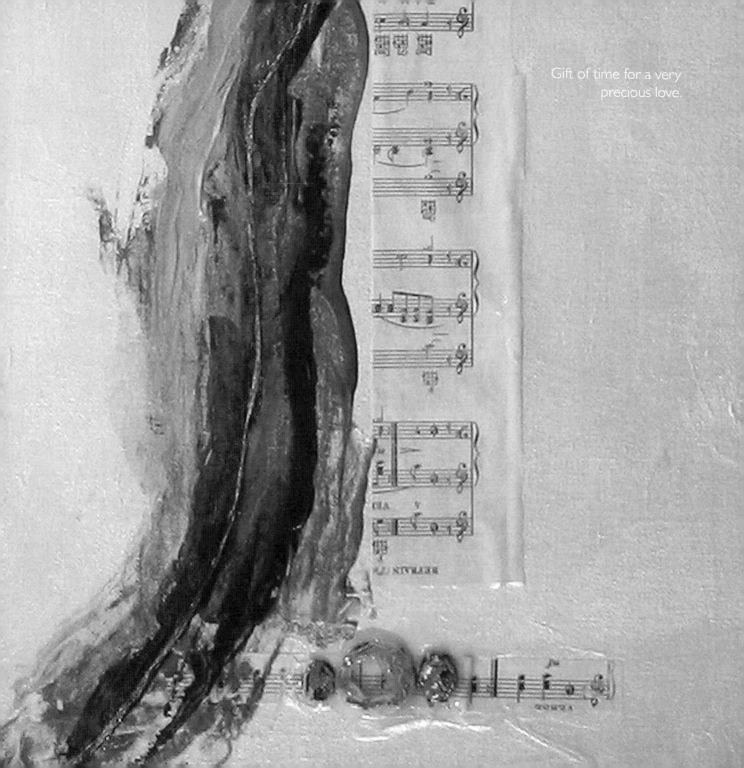

Gift of time for a very
precious love.

CHAPTER FIVE

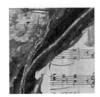

TEARS OF THE FATHERS, TEARS OF THE SONS

"...sorry for the tears, Fran. Momma has been gone thirteen years and when I remember
the pain and the anguish, I am once again overcome."
—*P. F. Hooper, M.D.*

Father of Juliarose

I noticed him in a group studying the gifts for sale on the silent auction table. He was handsome, graying, and walked with a slight limp. He waited until the people surrounding me had moved away before approaching, my book in his hand, leafing through the pages. I held out my hand and looked in his eyes.

"My daughter died from breast cancer last year," he said. His face showed so much pain, there were tears just at the back of his eyes. "I saw her just 3 months before her death. She knew she wasn't going to make it this time. Her mother called to tell me when Juliarose was gone. She was crying."

41

"I filled a void in Juliarose's life. She was about 3 years old when her mother and I married; she did not know her father and never saw him. I loved her so very, very much.

"When she married she moved to Dallas and lived there the rest of her life. She was a full-time energetic mother with four children, the oldest a son in West Point.

"Her first diagnosis of breast cancer came when she was 37. She opted for double mastectomy [one prophylactic] because she said she "wanted to nip it in the bud" and not worry about it any more."

He said with pride, "In 1999, she rode in the "Bike for Life" from California to Florida. This was before the recurrence."

He stopped, looked away, and choking, said, "After five years of remission came metastacized breast cancer."

He swallowed, "It took her life. And left me with this void in my life."

Image left and right: Gift of time for Dee. Caring spirit.

Tears of the Sons

"Our mother died of breast cancer. She suffered horribly.

"The first diagnosis was back about 1970. I guess she had a radical mastectomy. You know that wasn't discussed openly back then, among family and especially boys and men— even sons.

"Then she received chemotherapy, I think. Some of these details are unclear. My brother and sister and I don't remember much.. After her initial chemo, she was then diagnosed with cancer in another part of her body, but we were told it was a "primary cancer," not a recurrence or metastacized breast cancer. We were told her case was written up in a medical journal because of the multiples of primary cancers.

"Over the twenty years of different cancers, she attempted every treatment that was suggested, even new or experimental ones. She fought the cancers for as long as she had the money for the doctor and hospital bills.

"Odd thing, now that I look back. When her money was all gone, she died."

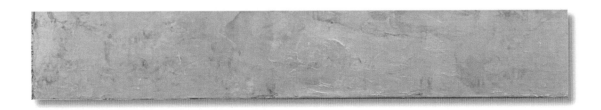

Eyes of Swedish Blue

"My mother has been diagnosed with cancer. She is such a wonderful and amazing woman. She has spent her whole life helping women with alcohol problems."

My friend is deeply saddened; I hear it in his voice and I see it in his eyes. By happenstance, my friend and I have Swedish heritage. His eyes are the Swedish blue like the eyes of our Swedish fathers.

"Ask your Mom her favorite color, so that I may paint for you a gift of time."

"She said her favorite color is the blue of my father's eyes."

Ah, yes, the blue I know so well. Images of Sweden's beauty and memories of blue eyes guided my hand across the canvas; the silvery beads and pearls stand for a lifetime of helping and giving.

Then from my soul I heard words like a poem, speaking as though aloud.

Eyes of Swedish blue…

…glow with love…

…glimmer with joy…

…glisten with tears.

And most of all, sparkle with humor.

No wonder this is Joan's favorite color!

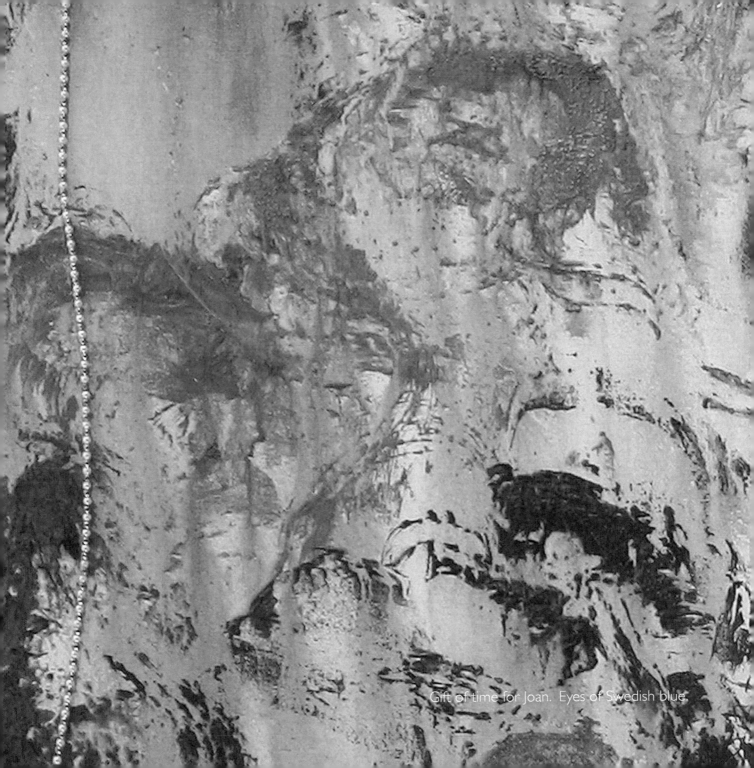
Gift of time for Joan. Eyes of Swedish blue.

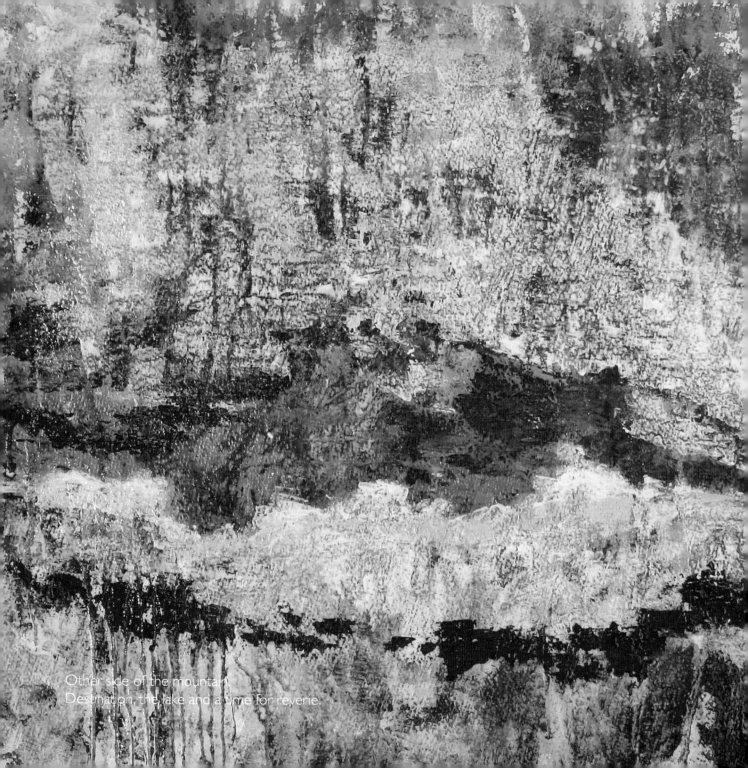

Other side of the mountain.
Destination, the lake and a time for reverie.

CHAPTER SIX

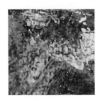

TAKE TIME FOR YOUR DREAMS

"Nothing happens unless first a dream…"
— Carl Sandburg

What Price Peace Of Mind?

Sheila had an aura of diffidence, and she seemed at first meeting somewhat shy. Her soft brown hair and smooth, clear skin made her seem younger than the mother of 15- and 17-year-old sons. Her most striking feature was the direct gaze of her deep blue eyes.

I was introduced to Sheila through a mutual friend who described her genetic situation of extreme risk for breast and ovarian cancer. He asked if I would be willing to meet and talk with her. Soon after our conversation, Sheila and I met for a glass of wine at a nearby restaurant after her office hours.

Slowly, calmly, Sheila shared the following details that profiled her 90% risk of developing breast cancer and 35% risk of developing ovarian cancer:

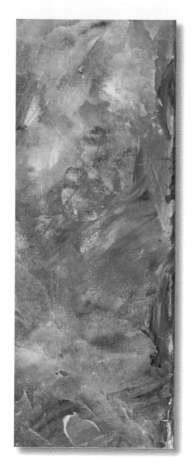

"My sister, Kay, was diagnosed with breast cancer when she was 32. She died from it when she was 36.

"My cousin, Lorri, (on my father's side), was diagnosed when she was 39 years old. We are all thankful that she has now been cancer-free for eleven years.

"Lorri's brother, Tom, was diagnosed with breast cancer when he was in his 40's. He is now cancer free. Again, we give thanks.

"After the genetics testing I consulted with physicians at M. D. Anderson. I've decided that I will have a bi-lateral mastectomy next month. Then after a couple of months I will have a hysterectomy and oophorectomy. The oophorectomy will eliminate the risk of ovarian cancer. I know that the bi-lateral mastectomy will not completely erase the risk of breast cancer, but it brings the risk down to a very small percentage."

Sheila paused a moment, then continued slowly, her voice even lower, "All of this seems so serious. But I consider it a gift that genetic research has made my family's cancer history a knowledge that allows me the choice of these surgeries. It can mean I may never have to endure the disease and the difficult chemo treatments. It can mean I can look forward to living for my kids and my grandkids. It is a gift of time, a gift of peace of mind."

As she spoke of these crossroads in her life I only nodded and waited for her questions.

I knew she was interested in my experience with bilateral mastectomy and in particular with my breast reconstruction – i.e.., was it immediate or delayed; what type of "replacement" did I opt for: self tissue, saline implants, or silicone implants. I also shared other patient's experiences that have been told to me. None of which, we both knew, were substitutes for the medical information from her physicians regarding her decisions.

Our discussion was as unemotional as though one were shopping for new kitchen appliances: what size, what finish, what warranties, how serviceable and for how long. I knew that the emotional reality would descend later, like an avalanche; even though she is prepared, even though she is grateful to have such a gift in this era of advanced medical knowledge. Even so, just as one must grieve for a loved one who passes away after a long, productive life, one must grieve for the amputation of one's womanhood. It is a part of the process and a part of the price of some peace of mind.

Later I called Sheila. "Sheila, I know you are going to have these surgeries, so that you 'can live for your kids and grandkids.' But be sure to 'live for yourself,' also. Take time for your dreams, Sheila."

"You know," she said, "I do have a dream. I want to someday travel through Europe."

Ah, yes, the gift of time.

Gift of time for Joan.

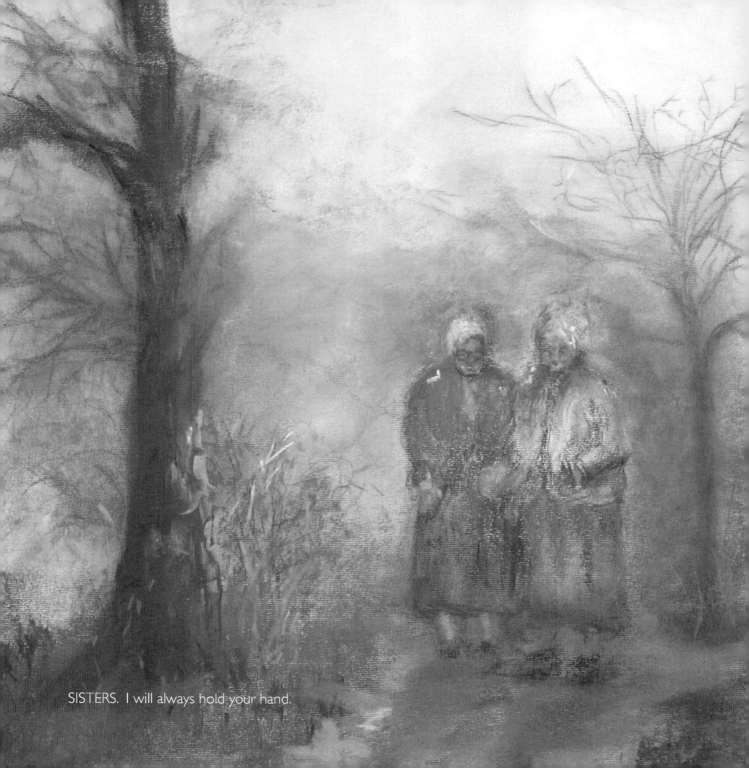

SISTERS. I will always hold your hand.

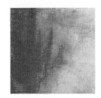

CHAPTER SEVEN

THE POWER OF EIGHT

Care, Share and Be Aware: The gold standard of support groups
Denise, Chris, and Rashel
Pam and Pat,
Joan, Linda and
one "mystery lady"

Care, Share and Be Aware:
The Power of Eight

"From the beginning we decided our group meetings would not be "pity parties.""

A decade ago eight women from all parts of the world, of all ages and different careers found they had a common denominator: breast cancer.

From Tehran, Iran to Orange, New Jersey; from Pittsburg, PA to Edinburg, Scotland; from New York City and Cumberland, Maryland, to El Paso, Texas. All were now in Houston; each was newly diagnosed and beginning treatment.

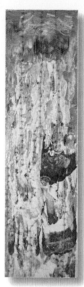

The youngest was 36. The oldest was 62.

They came from the fields of education and science, business and medicine.

Four were pre-menopausal; four were past menopause.

Two had subsequent recurrences.

Seven were white; one was black.

Five were later awarded BMW Hero of The Year, a recognition given to those in the breast cancer fields of medicine and advocacy.

Four volunteered for Reach for Recovery and two have continued their volunteer work for American Cancer Society.

One became the inspiration for a memorial resource library within the breast center.

For two years they nurtured their new organization, as one would nurture a child, determined that its value continue for those who were "brand newly diagnosed." It was an hour of good cheer, smiles, laughter and easy conversation in contrast to the sober, difficult hours of treatment for breast cancer. "We convinced our first nurse facilitator that she did not have to walk on eggshells around us after her gift of a folding hair brush, given to us who were chemo-bald was received with humor and chuckles. Someday the hair would return." One still keeps the brush in her purse every day.

The eight:

Linda, the first originator, a speech therapist whose students call her a "peach terrorist"

Chris, the woman with a way with words, whose recurrence prompted "My body has betrayed me!"

Rashel, the analytical, the "brain," had wanted to study medicine but was steered into geology and micro-paleontology.

Joan, the oldest of the 8, a hospital auxiliary volunteer.

Pat, a school nurse, with a wild and wacky sense of humor, ("if we had men in our support group imagine the possibilities".)

Pam, an elementary school teacher.

Denise, an x-ray technician, the youngest, the first to succumb, the inspiration for a memorial library.

The mystery woman who prefers anonymity, remains a mystery.

Gift of time for the lacemaker.

The Celebrations: From Borrowed Balloons To Boas

After two years, the group had grown to about 30 who regularly attended the monthly meetings – it was time to have a party – a celebration of life!

The first celebration of life was held in March. Spring time, the time of nature's renewal seemed symbolic. From then on, the celebration continued annually each March and "traditions" began, such as shrimp on the menu because the first party featured shrimp. For the first party there was no "theme." Decorations were balloons that had been left in the conference room by the party the night before. When Esther assumed the role of "nurse facilitator" for the support group, she became the "hostess with the most-est." And does Esther know how to "throw a party?" Whoooo-how, does she ever! There was a theme for each party. One year – rodeo roundup with hats, bandanas and barbecue. Another year – Hawaiian luau with leis; grass skirts for the brave, bright flowered shirts for the less brave, edible orchids on the tables. Last year "putting on the ritz" with hot pink feather boas on the survivors' shoulders, sexy, slinky with sequins the dress code. Next year: is a surprise to be announced.

Little wonder the invitation list is now over 300.

The "Pink Posse"

What, you ask, is a "pink posse?" It is Esther and Tosha and their "deputies," Jennifer, Vickey, Cynthia, Elaine (working from a wheelchair, and known as "the high sheriff" of the posse) wearing pink nurses' uniforms – zipping up and down the halls making the daily rounds.

It is the supporters who join the "chase," hunting and gathering leis and edible orchids, feather boas and sparkly, sequined posters announcing THIS IS A PARTY!

It is the "knitting ministry" and seamstresses who create comforting afghans and pillows for patients waking up from anesthesia.

It is the breast center staff and their friends who energetically search out and buy gifts to fill Esther's "Caring Closet," and the books for the memorial resource library.

It is the "prayer warriors" who stand by for special requests to comfort family and friends.

It is the nurses, doctors, survivors, friends who, with dedication, determination, and most of all with heart, carry on the tradition started by eight women.

It is all those who, like Esther, hope that at the end of life, what they have done will have made a difference.

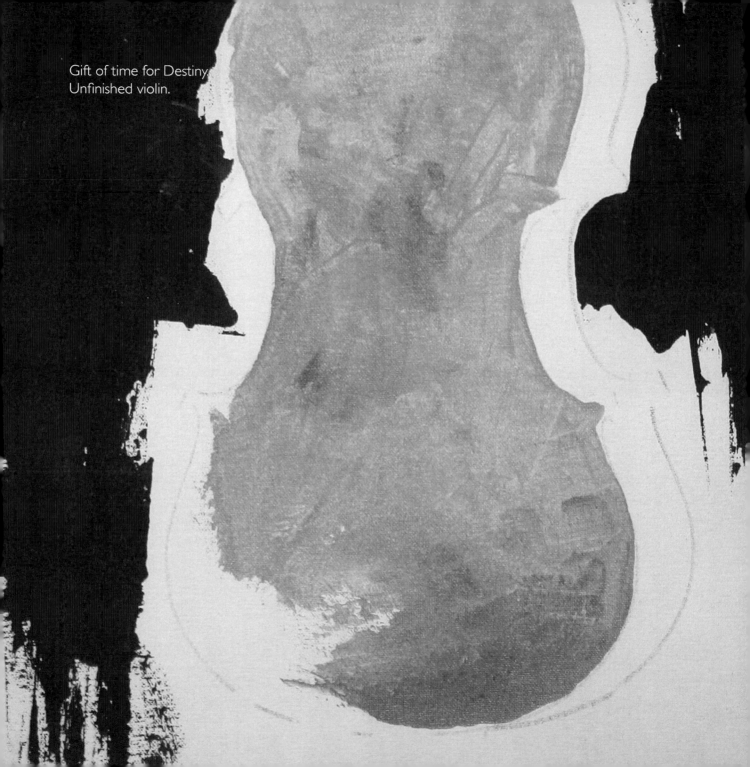

Gift of time for Destiny.
Unfinished violin.

CHAPTER EIGHT

TOO YOUNG

"You are a child of the universe, no less than the trees and the stars;
…and whether or not it is clear to you, no doubt the universe
is unfolding as it should.
Therefore be at peace with God, whatever you conceive Him to be…"
— From *Desiderata*, Max Ehrmann

Unfinished Violin. Unfinished Life

Her name is Destiny.

She has breast cancer.

She is 29 years old.

Some people have told me they think this vignette needs more detail. But, the other information I have about Destiny detracts from the powerful impact of: Name of Destiny and diagnosed with breast cancer at the age of 29. When you are 29 your life is "unfinished" – whether you go on to live lots more years or not.

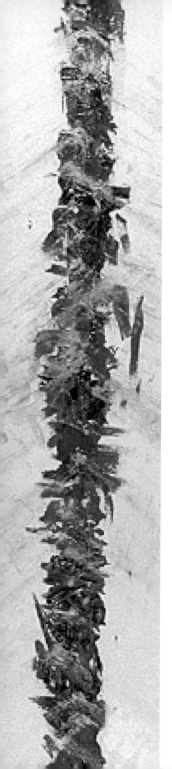

Stars for Jewels

A note came recently that read:

> "My best friend is Stephanie who is struggling with breast
> cancer. Would you paint for her? Her favorite color is red,
> plus she likes "jewel tones."

Sometimes red is difficult, a color too bold to allow a painterly composition. Jewel tones, though, imply gemstones. Rubies, sapphires, emeralds, topaz. Precious and semi-precious beauty from the earth, placed there by mother nature, dug and cut and polished by man, then surrounded by gold for rings and necklaces, bracelets and tiaras. Ornaments of value sometimes coveted, sometimes cherished.

The note continued:

> "Stephanie is a high school teacher. Her children are 10
> and 7 years old. She has had breast cancer less than a year.
> The treatments may not be successful. And she is only 36."

The next note came about two weeks later. "The treatments were not successful for Stephanie and she has succumbed."

Her son and daughter know she still watches over them and she will for as long as they live.

A mother's life whose love is cherished. Her ornaments now are angel wings with stars for jewels.

Dear God, I work for a cure.

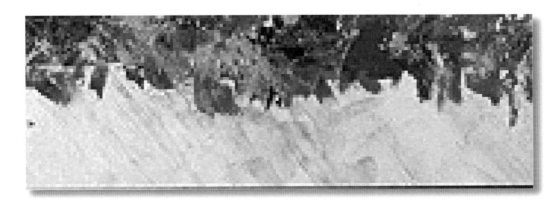

Image above and left: Gift of time for Stephanie. Stars for jewels.

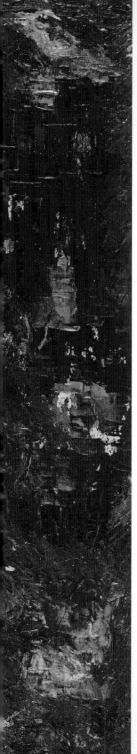

Four Victorias

"I am the third Victoria. My mother's name is Victoria. Her mother's name was Victoria. My daughter is now the fourth Victoria. How do we keep this all straight? And who answers when someone says 'Victoria?' Well, most people call me Vickie. My Mother answers sometimes to Victoria but mostly to "Mom." We call my daughter Ann because that is her second name."

"I love the color purple. Not the royal purple of queens, but the purple drama of nightclubs and spotlights on stages. The showy purple of Hollywood stars, with glitter and feathers. The atmospheric purple of twilight and storm clouds, of distant mountains reflected in silver water. The lush and heady purple of tropical gardens, orchids and bougainvillea."

"Breast cancer came when I was 39. Treatments are now over, but there were complications. Now my reconstructed left breast is scarred and lumpy. But no longer painful. And so far, cancer free."

"I give thanks for what is truly important: my breast is cancer free. And thanks for what is truly beautiful: mountains in twilight, gardens with orchids. And for four Victoria's — mothers and daughters — more reasons I am thankful."

Gift of time for Vicki. Purple's true beauty.

For Lisa

Care, Share and Be Aware meets the second Tuesday of each month. Beginning the meeting this January 9th,, Esther held up a large, colorful birthday card. "Tomorrow is Lisa's birthday. She isn't doing very well. Let's pass this around and everyone sign it with a love note for her." Everyone present knew that "not doing well" was code for time was getting short...

A midnight delivery in January.

"Diana," Esther telephoned, "can you come with me? It is getting late and dark, but tomorrow is Lisa's birthday, I have a card for her." It was not necessary to say more.

They agreed to meet because they were friends and co-workers, always supporting each other in the quest to share their loving concern with their breast cancer patients. A dark drive at midnight in January along unfamiliar streets, was just another day. The birthday card, a message of love, was left on Lisa's front door to be found the next morning.

A midnight rosary in February.

"I sat with Lisa until midnight," Esther told me. Tomorrow her husband will take her home to be comfortable these last few hours. And so she can be with her cats and with her art.

Lisa was not responsive, but Esther took her hand and said, "I don't have my rosary, Lisa, so I will use your hand." Touching Lisa's knuckles, Esther prayed the 'Our Fathers' and 'Hail Mary's.'

"Is Lisa Catholic?" I asked Esther.

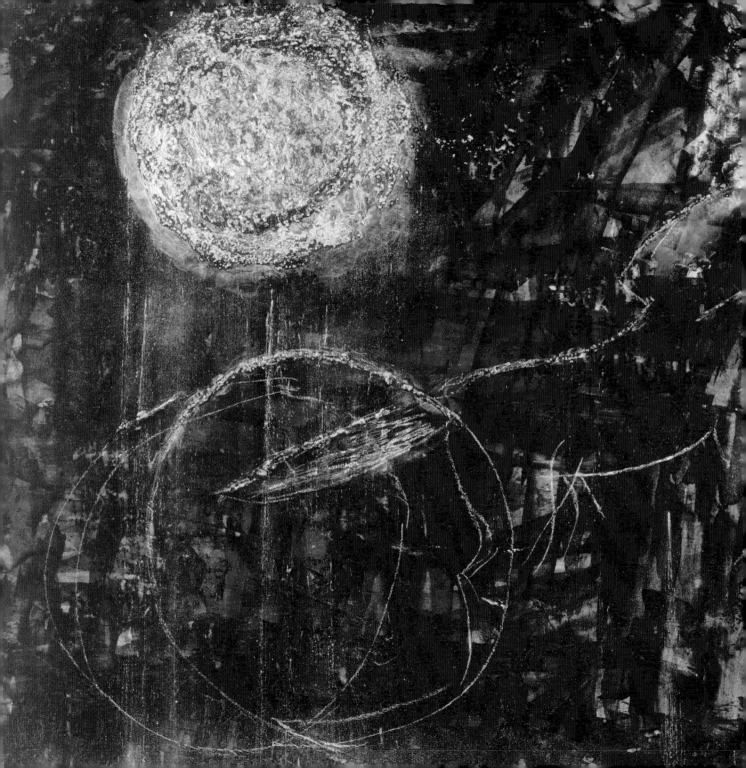

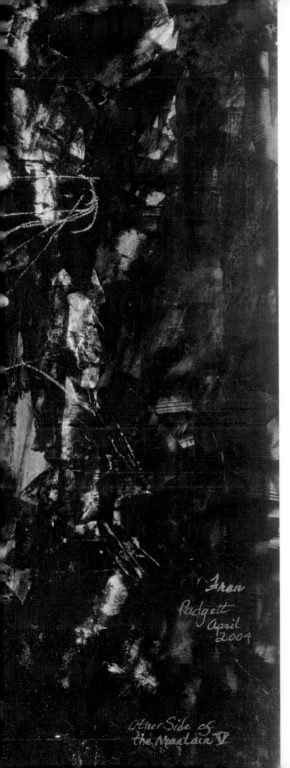

"I don't know," Esther replied softly, her eyes misty.

"You're right," I said in a whisper, "it doesn't matter."

Solace at midnight…still February

Esther nodded that it would be OK for Lisa's son to tenderly place her cats on the bed at her side. "Puffy," "Goober," and "Mo" curled next to her as they always had and kept their vigil until she entered the peace of eternity.

Other side of the mountain. Destination, the moon.
"We ran as if to meet the moon
That slowly dawned behind the trees …… "
from *Going for Water* by Robert Frost.

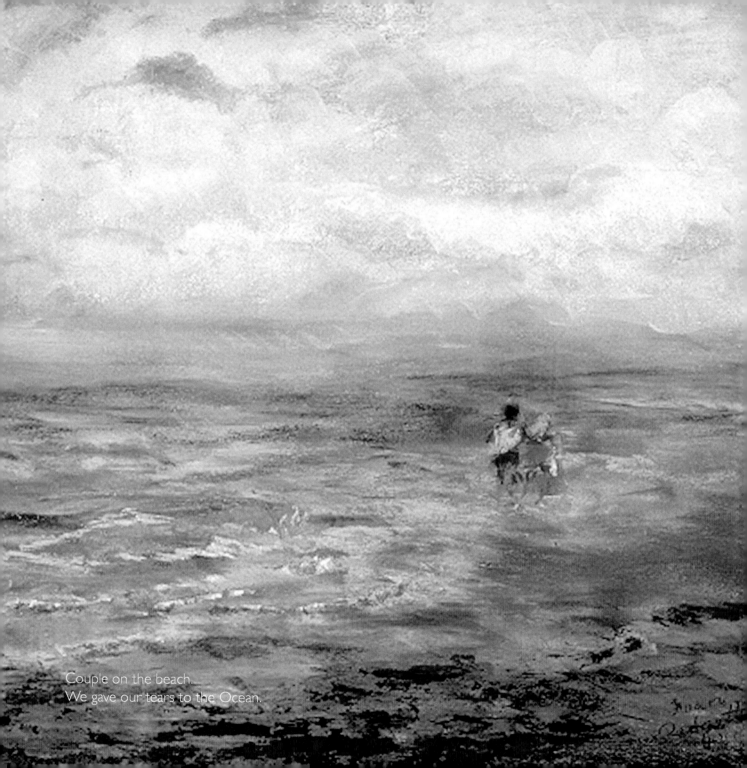

Couple on the beach.
We gave our tears to the Ocean.

CHAPTER NINE

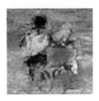

THE POWER OF LIFE SURVIVES

In this book are stunning stories of the power of life. A power that transcends traumatic cancer treatments. The power that overcomes shock when diagnosed at only twenty-nine years old. And the power that survives after death.

Anna: A Love Story

From Mark:

"While visiting our Houston Office from Chicago last week I had the joy of seeing your Exhibit. The piece Couple on the Beach struck a chord with me. My wife Anna succumbed to cancer last year. We visited the beach often and symbolically gave our tears to the Ocean. I would be interested in knowing the purchase price of the piece."

I am intrigued. "Struck a chord" is a musical analogy not expected in a man's writing. "Gave our tears to the Ocean," could have been written about fated and star-crossed lovers by an 18th century poet.

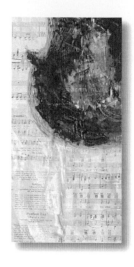

While we waited until the exhibit was over and the painting could be packed for transport, I called Mark. "Please tell me more about you and Anna."

"We had sixteen years crammed full. Those were wonderful years together.

"The beach where we walked in tears was Flagler Beach in Florida. We loved living near the ocean and enjoyed the beach when we were in San Diego and in Oregon. But we moved to Chicago for our careers and that is where I am now.

"Anna was born on nine-eleven. On nine-eleven-oh-one she turned 49. I was in Houston and was scheduled to fly back to Chicago for her birthday. With all planes grounded, I managed to find a rental car the next day to drive home. We didn't plan a party nor did I have a present. She met me at the rental car return with a picnic basket filled with sandwiches, cheese, a bottle of Merlot. We ate it in her car ("Cubby" I'll tell you about later) sitting in the parking lot.

"Anna liked to give a special name to everything in her life and she named her car "Cubby." It was a Jaguar roadster and when it was in our garage next to my car a Jaguar sedan, I guess it seemed like a baby.

"But she didn't name our Black Lab dog. I named her Anya. I said at least one female named Anna in this house is going to listen to me! We both laughed.

"Anna was everyone's teacher and befriended all types of people. She was a gardener and seemed to have a communion with the earth and with the sea.

She had studied Buddhism. She befriended the local group of Hell's Angels when we lived in San Diego. I know a lot of people are afraid of them. One day in Chicago after Anna was diagnosed and undergoing chemo, we heard this roar in the street just outside our house. Some of those Hell's Angels riders had heard she was sick and had come to see her. We both loved motorcycles and when we lived in Oregon we rode Harley-Davidson's.

"Nine-eleven-oh-two was Anna's 50th birthday – that was before she was diagnosed. We had a grand and glorious celebration. I had been in London and while there I found a sapphire and diamond ring and had it specially wrapped. She loved the ring. During the chemo treatments, when her body swelled we had the ring sized up; then when she lost weight, we had it sized down.

"The cancer was diagnosed in the spring of '03. I went with Anna for her chemo sessions. She always made them a picnic taking a basket lunch to help pass the time. We always got up early and listened to the classical music radio station. Then we would leave for those sessions that lasted for usually about six hours.

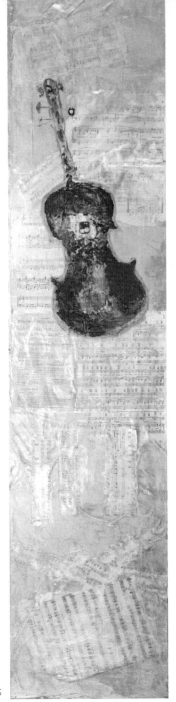

Image left and right: Gift of time for Anna. The power of her life survives

"Classical music was one of the many things we both loved. My degree is in Music from Appleton, Wisconsin. Even though she was a tomboy, she played violin for the Detroit Youth Symphony.

"The winter of '03-'04 she was often cold because of the chemo. She had a mink coat so we went to Marshall Fields and shopped for a hat. We found a mink hat but she wouldn't let me buy it for her unless I would agree to a new coat for myself.

"That night when she thought I was sleeping I watched her put on the hat and go prancing around the house looking at herself in all the mirrors.

Her birthday of nine-eleven-oh-three was to be her last birthday but of course we didn't know that then. Nor did we have a premonition – at least I did not. And then Christmas of 03 was her last Christmas, again no premonition.

"In the Spring of 04 she had lost a lot of weight and planned to shop for a new wardrobe. She was taking pain medication but declined hospice because she said she believed she would be surviving; but after she was gone I found a book she kept where she designated whom she wanted to have certain special belongings.

  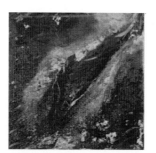 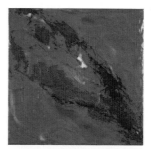

Above and left: from The gift of time suite for Eartha.

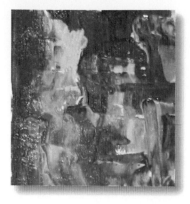

"We had two memorial services for Anna. The first one was in Chicago at German Lutheran church especially for her family. And then one at the Buddhist Center in Denver for her many friends

"Her circle of family and friends now communicate with each other by way of a special website. Her spirit keeps them energized and engaged."

When the exhibit was over, Couple on the Beach was prepared and packed, then shipped to Mark in Chicago. When he received it he called.

"I wanted to hang "Couple on the Beach" in the living room. But you know how paintings tell you where they want to be installed? It is now in the dining room near Anna's favorite painting "Dreamworks." An amazing thing. "Couple on the Beach" is now at the almost exact center of this house."

I wrote: "Yes, Mark, I am not surprised. Anna's spirit, the "power of her life survives" and has directed the placement of the image that struck the chord for you. Along with the memory of your combined tears to the Ocean, may you always find joy in having the painting."

Learn to read and you can learn everything else.
— Florence Helen Beatty Bowe

Becky: Peter Rabbit plus 6000 Gifts

Becky's house is filled with small gifts from hundreds of her students. Her shelves are filled with books. Her drawers are filled with notes and letters from her students. Her coffee table is stacked with the children's books she was planning to give to this year's students. Especially including Peter Rabbit. "Many of the important lessons in living can be taught from the stories of Peter Rabbit."

She was a specialist in reading recovery teaching elementary students who needed her. She "peopled" their lives with gentle animals like Flopsy and Mopsy, and youthful heroes and heroines like Rebecca of Sunnybrook Farm.

Forty-two years and six thousand kids. Six thousand youngsters who came to her for only a few hours. And in those few hours she influenced the rest of their lives because through reading they found the door to education opened. Sometimes they would leave their lives of misery and abuse to dwell a few enchanting hours in a beautiful story-book world. And many of "Becky's kids" found they could make a wondrous escape from a vicious cycle of poverty and neglect by starting a different life through the book avenue of education.

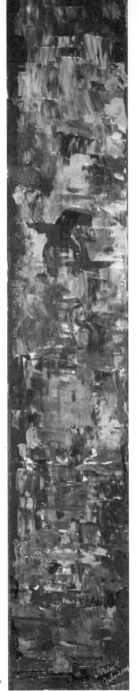

Image left and right: Gift of time for Becky. It was just a "blip."

Becky found within each child what was unique and good and special. No matter how "rascally" he might be, or petulant she might be. Every child should have at least one teacher like Becky. A teacher who accepts, and who praises, who teaches and rewards with books especially chosen as the one book that this newly reading youngster will cherish and remember and grow from.

Breast cancer was just a "blip" in Becky's school schedule. Starting with surgical biopsies of an unrelenting fibrocystic condition, through to finally an invasive ductal carcinoma. Through these years, all doctors' and hospital visits were scheduled for school holidays.

Once I stood with her family in the hall outside the operating room. As the gurney went by with Becky draped in white sheets, en route to the bright lights and surgeon, we could pat her arm. She looked so frail and afraid, there were tears on her cheeks. This was her first biopsy, done more than 30 years ago, when breast lumps were surgically excised in the hospital. As was routine at that time, she had agreed to the possibility of a mastectomy if the tissue was found malignant. Across the following thirty years, the biopsy routine varied and became less painful, less scary. But then cancer was detected in 2001 and her fears returned. True to her past, the lumpectomy was scheduled for the beginning of summer vacation, with the difficult (for her) radiation occupying all the weeks of the summer.

Six years after the diagnosis, she was once again preparing the school room to be ready for her next group of kids. Her family would joke: "Becky will never retire; she will teach forever." They didn't expect that to be prophetic, but last week she took her last breath while at school. Quickly, painlessly she was gone. Now she is a "teacher forever."

Her teacher friends are preparing a garden in her memory that will be on the grounds of the school where she taught. Without a doubt, Becky's kids, now grown might see "Peter Rabbit" peeking out from among the flowers.

A memorial garden is special. But a lifetime giving books, reading and knowledge is the power that survives.

I asked Becky's husband Bob to help me add up how many books she had given over the years. He said, "let me get my calculator." It wasn't an exercise in adding, but in multiplying. "Must be in the thousands," he said.

The following is excerpted from my dedication remarks for the unveiling of "Cove at Sunrise" at The Denise Veillon Memorial Library in The Breast Center at Houston Northwest Medical Center.

The Cove at Sunrise: A Secret Magic

"Once upon a time in my life before breast cancer, I was driving down a narrow country road. On a whim I turned right onto an even narrower road just to see where it might lead. On my left was a hill with dense woods. On my right was another little road sloping down toward the edge of the water. I parked, got out and walked over to a footbridge. Halfway across the bridge I stopped to look at the shallow water from both directions and I thought, how pretty, how peaceful. Feeling reflective, I left a few minutes later. I drove away not expecting to ever return.

"But a few years later, in my life after being diagnosed with breast cancer, I found myself drawn to drive that same narrow road just at dawn, and once again, found the turn to the right. When I came to the slope, I continued down to the water's edge, parked, and walked out onto the footbridge.

Other side of the mountain. Destination, the cove.

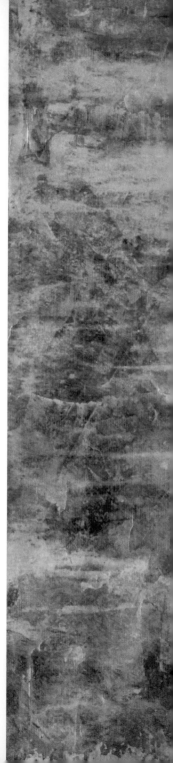

"The cove looked different to me this time. A little wooden sign told me this was "Wilhelmina's Cove." Looking across along one edge of the water, trees were reflected, creating dark shade.

"Looking down, almost directly under where I stood, lily pads circled out toward the center; lily pads not just of green, but of yellows and purples and deep burgundy, more beautiful than any Monet. The air was hushed; the only sounds were of small insects spinning and whirring. Then suddenly, flashing for a few moments of time, the atmosphere became shimmering with a brilliance only the power of the sun can create. A vision strengthening to my spirit, soothing to my soul.

"There is a secret and a magic about this cove! I believe it is why I was drawn to paint this enchanted place and this flashing instant of time.

"Wilhelmina's Cove is a real place. Wilhelmina was a real woman. She succumbed to breast cancer half a century ago. And I believe the beauty of the cove I saw in that instant, the brilliant golden sunrise, symbolizes the strength and spirit of breast cancer women of all time.

"Eveline, Linda, Rashel, Mary, Suzanne, Sharon, Roxanne, Anna, Sheridan, Brenda, Kathy, Chris, Vickey, Victoria, Tosha, Diane, Mary:

"As we live our lives of breast cancer recovery, MAY WE ALWAYS BE STENGTHENED BY THE SUNRISE, SOOTHED BY THE SUNSET, AND STRENGTHENED ONCE MORE AT THE NEXT SUNRISE."

Stopping by Woods on a Snowy Evening

Whose woods these are I think I know.

His house is in the village though;

He will not see me stopping here

To watch his woods fill up with snow.

My little horse must think it queer

To stop without a farmhouse near

Between the woods and frozen lake

The darkest evening of the year.

He gives his harness bells a shake

To ask if there is some mistake.

The only other sound's the sweep

Of easy wind and downy flake.

The woods are lovely, dark and deep,

But I have promises to keep,

And miles to go before I sleep,

And miles to go before I sleep.

— *Robert Frost*

Other side of the mountain. Rusty Bridge.
To a further destination.